Implant-Supported Prostheses: Occlusion, Clinical Cases, and Laboratory Procedures

DEDICATION

To my wife (Pepa) and my children
(Jaime, Silvia, David, and Pepita)
for all the stolen hours.
To my parents (Angeles and Vicente)
for the many unselfish hours they gave me.

Implant-Supported Prostheses: Occlusion, Clinical Cases, and Laboratory Procedures

Vicente Jiménez-López, MD, DDS

With Pedro Torroba Laviña, CDT

qb
quintessence
books

Quintessence Publishing Co, Inc
Chicago, Berlin, London, Tokyo, São Paulo, Moscow, Prague, and Warsaw

Library of Congress Cataloging-in-Publication Data
Jiménez-López, Vicente.
  [Prótesis sobre implantes. English]
  Implant-supported prostheses: occlusion, clinical cases, and laboratory
  procedures / Vicente Jiménez-López: co-author, Pedro Torroba Laviña.
  p. cm.
  Includes bibliographical references and index.
  ISBN 0-86715-257-5
  1. Implant dentures. I. Torroba Laviña, Pedro. II. Title.
  [DNLM: 1. Dental Prosthesis--atlases. 2. Dental Implantation--atlases.
  WU 17 J61p 1994a]
  RK667. I45J5513 1995
  617.6'92--dc20
DNLM/DLC
for Library of Congress
                           94-34517
                             CIP

quintessence
books

Editor: Adam Haus

Composition: Grafisches Atelier Michael Gradias, Wolfenbüttel
Design: SPAINFO, S.A.-Madrid
Printing and binding: Gráficas Monterreina, S. A., Madrid
Printed in Spain

FOREWORD

Predictable long-term clinical success with osseointegrated prosthetic substitutes for teeth, whether replacing a single tooth or the entire dentition in a patient with severe resorption of the maxilla and mandible, requires careful consideration of how to adapt and apply prosthetic materials, components, and procedures in a situation in which experience from conventional prosthodontic methodology cannot be directly relied upon, since the biological conditions are definitely different.

Topographical precision resulting in avoidance of stress is a prerequisite, even if the load-carrying integrating bone, because of its elasticity, provides a certain resilience, and even if its remodeling capacity can compensate for some surgical and prosthetic inadequacies. Still, utmost precision of the design of the prosthetic superstructure should be aimed at.

It is equally important to consider how to make the masticatory system accept these constructions, to allow for harmonious integration in the neuromuscular functional complexities.

Creative thinking based on clinical observations and trials, followed by careful adaption of new procedures to existing experience and technical protocols, is needed.

Dr. Jiménez-López has approached his topic according to this philosophy. He has contributed a meticulously developed, innovative, and detailed solution for safe and reliable prosthetic rehabilitation of the edentulous patient, considering the entire spectrum of requirements from anchorage to esthetics.

Therefore, this book is useful not only for those specialists who provide this particular kind of treatment, but also those in daily dentistry when the edentulous patient is examined and evaluated, and different treatment modalities are considered.

This book facilitates the correct identification of those patients who would benefit from osseointegrated oral reconstructions, and offers solutions for optimal clinical treatment.

P-I Brånemark
Professor, MD PhD ODhc ScDhc ahc FDSRCS
Gothenburg

PREFACE

In the 1980s we witnessed the birth of a new specialty, osseointegrated implantology.

We were fortunate to witness this "public birth" and to contribute new clinical and prosthodontic techniques that will be described in this book. All this was possible thanks to Professor Brånemark, who undoubtedly has been the most important figure of modern dentistry. I feel the most sincere respect, admiration, and affection for Dr. Brånemark.

In 1980, while expanding my postgraduate studies at the University of Southern California, I came in contact with the world of implants for the first time. At that time we were taught to avoid implant treatment because of the high failure rate with the nonosseointegrated techniques. Only on few occasions were subperiosteal implants recommended.

I had the chance to know and appreciate the late Professor Donald Curnutte while sharing mornings in his 3 x 3 meter office full of books and papers. At the time he was "Occlusion Chairman"; his passing away was a great loss to the profession. His warm, humane, and fatherly voice would help me solve my doubts that through my youth and inexperience I brought before him.

The afternoons I spent in Dr. Albert Solnit's office, a great theoretician and clinician, who invited me over just because I was from Spain (a country he adores), helped me to learn how to relate his knowledge to everyday prosthodontic practice.

I would like to remember the many people I met during those years I spent specializing.

Among them, good old Dr. Stuart, who, despite his age, had the vigor of a 20-year-old and who radiated science through his teachings (we miss you).

Professor Erik Martínez Ross, who welcomed me to Mexico with the affection proper of a master of occlusion. On my first day he said something that has been very important to my career: "Anyone who crosses the Atlantic to learn deserves all my support." I have tried to reciprocate with those who have visited me. He taught me many things, and the last time we met a few months ago he bid me farewell saying "te quiero mucho" (I love you very much). How hard it is to show these feelings between men; you have to be a great man to do so.

Professor Solberg, who opened the doors of the Occlusion Department at UCLA for me. Through him I learned that the TMJ is one more of the body joints and should be treated as such.

Later on, I was fortunate enough to have as dear friends two of the true genuises in temporomandibular dysfunction: Professor Tore Hansson (University of Amsterdam and St. Joseph's Hospital, Phoenix, Arizona), who is all kindness, affection, and gentleness, one of the people who has greatly researched and contributed to this field, and who gave me the opportunity to participate in his book Craniomandibular Dysfunction; *and Professor Sandro Palla (University of Zurich) whose earnest work hides an affable, intimate, open personality, and a good friend of his friends. Through them, I learned the multidisciplinary approach to treating the stomatognathic system.*

Dr. Guillermo Román, who practices in Los Angeles, aided me in learning the importance of esthetics in implant-supported prostheses. Despite his youth, he is candid, kind, and dedicated to his friends.

Last, but not least, is my mentor Dr. José Luis Lopez Alvárez. He has not only taught me dentistry, but through his exemplary character I have learned the principles and ethics that guide my private and professional life. I have tried to imitate you in both of these areas, but I doubt I have ever achieved it!

To all those I have forgotten unintentionally, I wish to express my gratitude and ask to be forgiven. I wish to thank all of those colleagues who attended my lectures or came to my office for advice. They awakened my own inquisitiveness and I learned much through their questions.

Vicente Jiménez-López

CONTENTS

CONTENTS

INTRODUCTION

THE PROSTHODONTIST

The role of the prosthodontist is very important in selecting, guiding, and offering solutions to the patient. He or she must:

(1) Perform an in-depth radiological study (panoramic radiograph and tomography) to evaluate which edentulous areas are adequate for implants.

(2) Consider which remaining teeth can be kept during treatment planning.

(3) Inform the surgeon as to the desired implant location for the best prosthodontic results. Teamwork requires that the surgical difficulties be discussed in advance so as to decide where to place the implants.

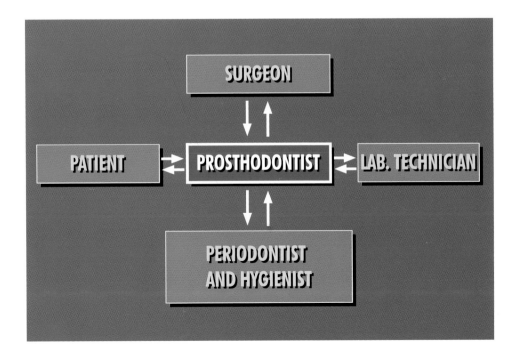

After implant osseointegration, the prosthodontist selects the preferred abutments in each case, depending on arch position, inclination, and opposing dentition.

In a later phase, and in close comunication with the laboratory technician, he or she will study and direct the construction of the prosthesis, always searching for adequate balance between esthetics, function, and hygiene.

Finally he or she will periodically evaluate the patient's occlusion, parafunction, stomatognathic system (TMJ, muscles, etc), and implants (bone resorption, pockets, etc), in communication with the periodontist and hygienist.

Characteristics of the Implant-Supported Prosthesis

In implant-supported prosthetics, the patient must be offered what is best for him or her. In the early stages of osseointegrated implantology, function and hygiene prevailed over prosthesis esthetics. Today, it is impossible to plan a dental prothesis without considering esthetics at the same level as hygiene and function. This is why in prosthodontic solutions multiple possibilities have been introduced, with the goal to have the three factors go hand in hand to offer the patient a state-of-the-art final result. All of them will be described in this book.

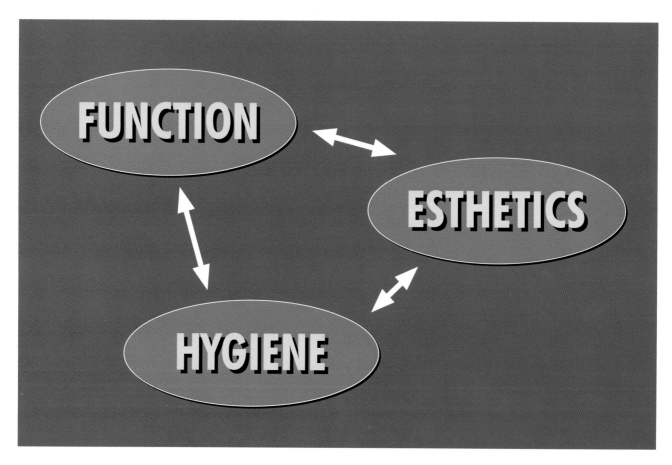

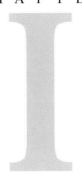

TREATMENT PLANNING

We have discussed the importance of initially communicating with the surgeon. Once the radiographic study (panoramic and tomography of the edentulous area) has been performed we will analyze various parameters to choose between a fixed or removable prosthodontic solution.

1.1 Remaining bone

Recent surgical advances (regeneration and osseous stimulation, as well as grafting) permit us at this time to place implants despite the existence of little remaining bone. There is no doubt that this has been a great achievement, since the number of patients that can benefit from osseointegration and fixed solutions has increased.

1.2 Number of abutments

A) Mandible

If it is possible to have good implant length, the minimum number of implants necessary for fixed solutions is four.

However, if the number of implants is increased, equally distributing them, better force distribution can be achieved.

Problems will surface if any of them fail; consequently, six to eight is the ideal number of implants to distribute fulcrums and foresee possible future losses due to problems of osseointegration.

B) Maxilla

If bone quality is good, the minimum number of implants necessary for fixed solutions is five or six.

Obviously, eight implants is better, if two distal implants can be placed in the pterygoid process. In extreme cases, one can increase the number of abutments. For removable prostheses, two implants is the minimum, although in many cases it is insufficient should implant failure occur. Here we have a large fulcrum that, even though it is beneficial, can prove to be uncomfortable and decrease patient masticatory function.

1.3 Masticatory function

The choice between an overdenture (upper and lower) or a fixed prosthesis depends on sufficient implant units for a fixed solution (more than four or five implants) and the patient's financial situation. In any event and following Dr. López Alvarez's techniques, as described in his book *Laboratory Techniques*, and referring to natural dentition, we shall describe the combinations possible. It must be remembered that fixed implant-supported prostheses lack resiliency. Conversely, overdentures are partially supported by soft tissues, so therefore are resilient.

Best results during mastication are achieved by opposing teeth that are fixed nonresilient prostheses. Included in this group is the natural dentition acting as opposing teeth.

A second solution that is acceptable for chewing efficiency is if one set of opposing teeth is fixed and the other resilient. Cases of implant-supported overdentures against opposing natural dentition are included here.

The worst situation is when both are resilient, which results in decreased chewing efficacy. Implant-supported overdentures against an opposing full denture are included here.

Whenever possible, the best treatment choice will be fixed prostheses in both arches.

If this is not possible, it is preferable to have a fixed lower prosthesis and an upper overdenture, because the lower will be a hybrid prosthesis that achieves a passive fit over the implants (see the technique of cylinders cemented to screw-type prosthesis, chapter IX) and lip height will allow us to leave the implants accessible for better patient hygiene.

1.4 Occlusal surfaces

According to the writings of Roman M. Cibirka (1992), no significant differences were found on implant force absorption (load) when gold, porcelain, or acrylic-resin occlusal surfaces were used.

In a certain way, this study questions the theory of "progressive implant loading," installing first a temporary fixed acrylic-resin prosthesis and, after a few months, substituting it for one in porcelain.

We believe that this is not necessary. We only place a provisional prosthesis in anterior teeth or when the removable prosthesis cannot be adapted to the healing caps (see chapter XI).

In upper and lower overdentures and lower hybrid prostheses, acrylic-resin teeth are used. In single and partial prostheses and in upper restorations we employ porcelain. Bruxists on occasion require metal occlusal surfaces.

In any case, we are open to exchanging acrylic resin for porcelain depending on the nature of the opposing dentition.

1.5 Esthetics

To obtain a good result, the smile line, tooth length, implant position, nasolabial angle, nasogenial sulcus, midline, etc, must always be considered.

All of these can be modified using various abutments and their specific techniques. We can also utilize removable rigid gingiva, as will be discussed later.

The esthetic factor will rarely, or never, determine fixed-prosthesis or overdenture selection.

1.6 Occlusion

It can be a determining factor in treatment choice. This will be described in chapters II, III, and IV.

1.7 Unfavorable prognoses

There are diseases that affect osseointegration adversely, such as diabetes, grave hepatic alterations, etc.

In general, these are related to the microcirculation regeneration process during osseous integration. They are not necessarily absolute contraindications, but because of the worst prognosis, the patient must be informed. Beware of psychiatric patients and heavy smokers!

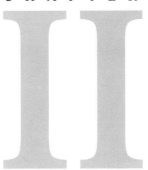

OUR PHILOSOPHY OF
IMPLANT-SUPPORTED PROSTHESES

2.1 Long-term results

For many years, the main goal in dentistry was to increase the longevity of teeth.

This belief has changed in the last few years after observing the good results achieved with osseointegrated implants, in our case with the Brånemark System. Long-term planning is necessary with every patient, taking into consideration not only future tooth loss near the implants but also alternative solutions in case we should lose implant osseointegration; all of this will influence the number of implants placed and possible modifications of the prosthesis, eliminating the need to construct a new one.

For example, if a certain case can be treated with two implants, three are preferred, because in case of a failure the same prosthesis can be supported by the two remaining implants. In this way we help the patient by reducing surgical anxiety and the risk, though small, of undergoing surgery with local anesthesia, analgesia, and in extreme cases general anesthesia.

2.2 Avoid implant overloading: passive fit

One of our main concerns has been, and is, implant overloading.

Considering a situation in which the fit of an implant-supported prosthesis is not fully passive, tensional forces develop over the implants and can lead to bone reduction around them, which in the long run may cause implant loss or at least reduce implant life expectancy.

Due to the design of the implant-prothesis complex with one flat surface against another, if we do not obtain a 100% fit, overloading will ensue.

For this reason, we consider it mandatory to achieve an absolutely passive fit over the implants. Reaching this goal is difficult because prosthesis construction is fairly complex.

In general, when casting, curved structures should be avoided due to the distortions that occur. We have developed the system of cemented cylinders over screw-retained prostheses (see chapter IX). This avoids the tensions produced due to the lack of passive fit in "hybrid prostheses." In fixed prostheses, we try to avoid splinted curved structures, which we break up through the use of attachments, converting them into three straight structures (see chapter X).

2.3 Equilibrated occlusion

It is indispensable to consider the occlusion, not only for patient comfort and better chewing efficiency, but to prevent excessive implant loading.

As a general rule, mutually protected occlusion is used, having maximum intercuspation coinciding with centric relation and anterior guidance during disocclusion in excursive movements (central incisors, lateral incisors, and canines, or all of them as a group). We thus avoid posterior tooth contact in all excursions (this is described in detail in chapter III).

To support the corresponding guides in the anterior group, we select the implants with better prognosis because of their length and situation in the arch.

2.4 The implant and the stomatognathic system

When dealing with implant-supported prostheses, one should not forget that we are working within a stomatognathic system that requires a series of general considerations:

A) Vertical dimension

If the vertical dimension is not physiological, it is causing an anatomical alteration of the patient's muscular system. If the vertical dimension is reduced, the length of the muscles is shortened during occlusion. At the same time, it influences facial esthetics, producing the typical "Popeye" face.

B) Bruxism

It is well known that bruxism is a form of eliminating internal tension and is often a cause of tooth loss.

Even though malocclusion can favor the appearance of this parafunction, there is a strong interrelationship between the central nervous system and stress. Bruxism is very common in the twentieth century (one of the more characteristic pathologies is known as the "urban syndrome").

Consequently, the appearance of these destructive habits must be avoided, and should they appear, nocturnal occlusal splints should be used to restrict the destructive effects of overloading. The patient must also be instructed on the noxious effect of clenching and grinding, so as to avoid the habits they are frequently unaware of.

In many cases, these patients are individuals with great masseter and temporal muscle mass. Their masticatory forces surpass the average, making bruxism a contraindication for implants according to some authors. This is not necessary in our opinion, but we are extremely careful during prosthesis fabrication for bruxing patients. Frequent occlusal follow-ups are mandatory, eliminating prematurities and interferences, as well as verifying good guidance in the anterior teeth. Nocturnal occlusal splints may also be employed.

C) Other habits and parafunctions

Several years ago, one of our patients periodically returned to our office with a fractured lower central incisor from his hybrid prosthesis over five implants.

Our concern for the case made us change the design of our metal structures. We thought the problem was at the metal-resin interface. After six months of multiple repairs, we opted for a new prosthesis with a different design. A month later the patient was back in the office with the same broken tooth. This time he was accompanied by his brother, who privately told us "the secret": the bearer of the prothesis used to open up Coca-Cola bottles with his mouth to show his friends the efficiency of his implants. We had not asked about parafunctions!

To avoid this, we must always be informed about abnormal habits and we must try to correct them. On many occasions, the success of the prosthesis will depend on a thorough history.

D) TMJ and muscles

This section deserves special attention.

When deciding on the treatment plan for an oral rehabilitation, and more so when dealing with an implant-supported prosthesis, we must consider the masticatory muscles and all the components of the temporomandibular joint (TMJ).

Natural teeth possess certain resilience that, on occasion, is a safeguard from advanced degenerative pathologies of the TMJ.

This will rarely be the case in implant-supported prostheses. Special attention must be given to the stomatognathic system as a whole. As a general rule, it must fulfill the following requirements:

— Muscular relaxation.
— Absence of articular inflammation.
— Condyle in stable position in centric relation.
— Adequate vertical dimension.
— Organic occlusion with anterior guidance and absence of interferences and prematurities.
— No pain present in any of the system's components.

Because in most cases, the patient has not had a stable prosthesis, with an acceptable occlusion and adequate vertical dimension, in place for years the centric relation bite record is difficult to obtain due to a lack of good muscle relaxation. When constructing a provisional prosthesis, it is very important to consider this and to take extra care in the final prosthesis; otherwise, we could convert the patient into a future TMJ patient.

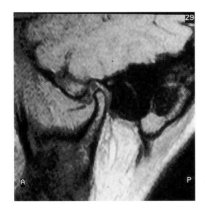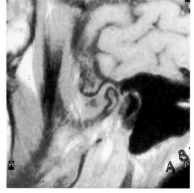

Magnetic resonance imaging (MRI) of condyle in the glenoid fossa with closed mouth. At left, the disk is in correct position with respect to the condyle and the posterior portion of the corresponding articular eminentia. At right, the disk is forward and irrestorable. (Courtesy of Dr. Carlos Benito.)

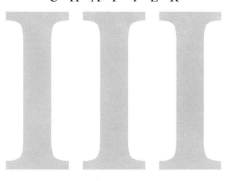

OCCLUSION

3.1 Introduction

Mandibular closure is very important, functionally speaking, because it ends with the contact of teeth from the upper and lower arches. To avoid iatrogenic damage to the stomatognathic system, it is important to consider the principles of occlusion.

Prosthesis design, which is sometimes underrated in implantology, will be important for the future prognosis of the installed appliance. Implants will not always be perfectly positioned, which will hinder our task in arranging tooth contacts correctly.

In general, we look for a prosthesis with an occlusion where maximum intercuspation coincides with the position of condylar centric relation.

Now we will define the basic principles of occlusion:

A) Centric relation

This is the physiological position of the condyles when they are centered in the fossae in their uppermost position and related correctly with the meniscus against the posterior incline of the articular eminence.

The successful introduction of the term meniscus into the definition of centric relation is a sign of openness within the occlusal philosophies. However, those clinicians who regularly treat patients with dysfunctional TMJ problems frequently observe that the meniscus is poorly placed, and in MRI studies it is seen ahead of the condyle. On few occasions is its physiological position restorable. This is partially due to this condition being totally asymptomatic, in many cases, presenting clinically with reciprocal clicks of variable intensity, which are painless and which sometimes go undetected by the clinician.

For this reason, we are inclined to believe that in the future centric relation will be referred to as the physiological position of the condyles in the fossae, eliminating overloads in the closed position over soft tissues, which will prove useful in preventing advanced lesions.

In any event, to achieve better communication with the readers, we shall still consider centric relation as the ideal physiological condylar position.

B) Maximum intercuspation

This is the tooth position where maximum occlusal contacts exist in the active chewing cusps (lower buccals and upper linguals) in relationship with the opposing teeth.

What we pursue in ideal occlusion is to have both positions (centric relation and maximum intercuspation) coincide. Maximum tooth contact does not interfere with the correct condyle position.

C) Working condyle and working side

When the mandible moves laterally, the (working) condyle on the side to which the jaw moves (working side) carries out an almost pure rotation on a vertical axis without any lateral displacement. Should a lateral displacement occur, a Bennett movement would be present.

D) Nonworking condyle and nonworking side

These are the opposite condyle and side of the working condyle and side. The condyle travels forward, downward, and medially, depending on the presence or absence of the Bennett movement variations that may exist.

E) Bennett movement

The Bennett movement is a full mandibular sideshift in which the working-side condyle will initially travel out from the glenoid fossa, later being able to move upward, downward, forward, backward, or a combination of these.

These changes in condylar position during lateral movements greatly influence occlusal anatomy, giving place to variations in cusp height, groove and incline positioning, as well as the lingual aspect of the upper anterior segment.

The Bennett movement does not always appear during lateral excursions. On occasion, it must be induced, and in other cases, it does not exist.

The Bennett induction maneuver is done by forcing the mandibular angle on the nonworking side towards the working condyle, producing on this side an outward sideshift, when the TMJ allows this to occur. This induction maneuver should be done on both sides while exploring lateral excursions of the mandible.

This covers the possibility that when the patient is sleeping on his/her side he or she could start a grinding parafunction. Since we foresee this situation, with the sideshift induction at the time of occlusal equilibration we can introduce adequate grooves that will allow an escape route for opposing cusps.

The Bennett movement takes place through different mechanisms. At this time, it seems that its presence is related to TMJ pathology, especially to hyperlaxitudes, whether or not they have an occlusal origin.

Since most implant patients have lost a great deal of teeth, leading to joint overloading, we should pay special attention to the Bennett movement when adjusting the occlusion.

F) Anterior disocclusion guide

In the ideal occlusion, we would like strong contacts in maximum intercuspation in the posterior teeth (molars and premolars) and softer contacts in the anterior teeth (canines, lateral and central incisors); once eccentric movements (lateral or protrusive) begin, the anterior teeth immediately become the guidance, disoccluding the posterior teeth.

The anterior guide should be as flat as possible allowing for posterior disocclusion. In this way, the whole system will function in harmony, avoiding unwanted TMJ tension originating from the occlusion.

As a general rule, a condylar sideshift of 3 mm should have a 1.5-mm separation in the opposing teeth on the nonworking side and a 1-mm separation on the working side.

If we follow these principles, overloading of the structures that keep the condyle in the articular fossa and of the anterior implants will not occur. This is due to the fact that the lingual aspects of the canines, laterals, and centrals will be in harmony with the inclination of the articular eminence, permitting physiological function of the stomatognathic system. It should

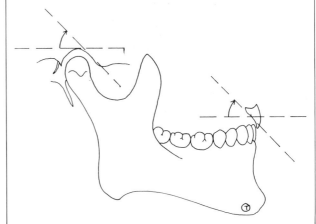

Fig. 3.1

Relationship between the inclination of the eminence and lingual aspect of the anterior segment.

be noted that because of the osseous anatomy of the anterior maxillary area, implant inclination will be similar to that of the eminence.

When developing the occlusion in a restoration, the anterior guide must be created first; once it is perfectly incorporated, we move on to adjust the occlusion in the posterior.

G) Posterior occlusal anatomy

The construction of posterior occlusal anatomy consists of correctly positioning cusps, fossae, and pathways, while searching for tooth-to-tooth and cusp-to-fossa relationships.

In the maxillary arch, the active cusps are the linguals:

— First and second premolars (one active cusp)... lingual cusp

— Molars (two active cusps)... mesiolingual and distolingual cusps

In the mandibular arch, the active cusps are the buccals:

— First and second premolars (one active cusp)... buccal cusp

— Molars (three active cusps)... mesiobuccal, distobuccal, distal cusps

The buccal cusps in the maxillary arch are nonactive:

— First and second premolars (one cusp)... the buccal

— Molars (two cusps)... mesiobuccal and distobuccal

The lingual cusps are nonactive in the mandibular arch:

— First and second premolars (one per tooth)... the lingual

— Molars (two per tooth)... mesiolingual and distolingual

The nonactive cusps participate in fossae configuration and bolus retention during mastication.

To achieve proper occlusion and efficient masticatory function, the active cusps must have their corresponding opposing fossae.

Distribution of active cusps with their corresponding fossae is done in the following way:

— Upper active cusps (lingual)

First upper premolar... distal fossa of the lower first premolar
Second upper premolar... distal fossa of the lower second premolar

Upper molars:

Mesiolingual cusp to central fossa of the opposing mandibular molar
Distolingual cusp to distal fossa of the opposing mandibular molar

— Lower active cusps (buccal)

First lower premolar... mesial fossa of first upper premolar
Second lower premolar... mesial fossa of second upper premolar

Lower molars:

Mesiobuccal cusp to mesial fossa of the opposing maxillary tooth
Distobuccal cusp to central fossa of the opposing maxillary tooth
Distal cusp to distal fossa of the opposing maxillary tooth

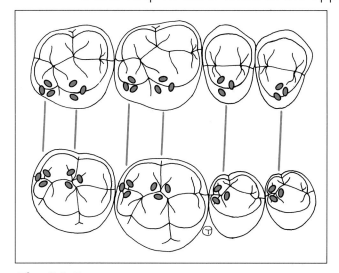

Fig. 3.2-A

Occlusion of the upper active cusps (lingual) into their corresponding opposing lower fossae.

Fig. 3.2-B

Occlusion of the lower active cusps (buccal) into their corresponding opposing upper fossae.

In this way we have arranged the cusps and fossae of the posterior component of the occlusion.

The next step will be to relate the cusp within the fossa. Some philosophies of occlusion support tripodization, while others prefer that the cusp tip contact the bottom of the fossa. Our philosophy is to seek cusp contact on the fossa incline. We try to obtain one, two, or three contact points, making sure they are really contact points and not surface contacts. Three contacts per cusp is considered the ideal situation but is seldom achieved. We do not believe that the cusp tip should be at the fossa's bottom, because to avoid lateral contacts, the active part will probably be very small. Considering that we can relate 38 cusps to 38 fossae, we believe that this is enough to obtain adequate masticatory function, even if we only achieve one contact in each fossa. This means we would have at least two in premolars (corresponding to one cusp and one fossa) and five in molars (cusps and fossae), which would give sufficient occlusal stability.

Now we have the cusps seated in the fossae (with point-like contacts), the condyle in centric relation, the absence of prematurities, and disocclusion through good anterior guidance. The

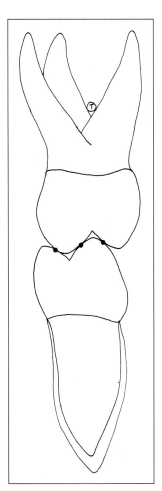

Fig. 3.3
Diagram of the active masticatory area.

grooves that will allow the cusps to exit from their fossae during working, nonworking, and protrusive movements are now designed.

Working (rotation and perhaps outward or other combinations) and nonworking (downward, forward, and medial) condylar movement must be considered for groove inclination and direction that will permit, according to the different mandibular movements, the cusps to exit their fossae without posterior contacts.

Evidently, the exit routes of the cusps follow their corresponding grooves, that is, the fossae exit paths are completely opposite in the upper and lower teeth.

Upper arch:

Working groove:	transversal towards buccal
Nonworking groove:	oblique towards mesial and lingual
Protrusive groove:	towards mesial

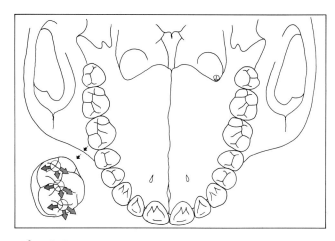

Fig. 3.4
Diagram of maxillary exit paths.
• Red → nonworking
• Blue → protrusive
• Green → working

Fig. 3.5
Diagram of mandibular exit paths.

Lower arch:

Working groove: transversal towards lingual
Nonworking groove: oblique towards distal and buccal
Protrusive groove: towards distal

It should not forgotten that all fossae need grooves to allow cusp exit without interferences. In Figs. 3.4 and 3.5 only one upper and lower tooth have been shown, but the direction of all grooves is similar in the rest.

In lateral excursions, this will only allow anterior tooth contact, while the posterior teeth remain completely free. However, in closure, only the posterior teeth will be in contact (cusps in fossae), the anterior teeth remaining almost free of contact.

The forces applied on the implants will be vertical with respect to the axis of the posterior teeth, thus avoiding loads on the anterior teeth.

H) Prematurities

Prematurities represent any tooth contact during mandibular closure, with the condyles in centric relation, that occurs before maximum intercuspation.

Prematurities force the condyles out of centric relation. If there are parafunctions, this can lead to articular and muscle overloading, as well as alterations of masticatory dynamics conducive to pathology in the long run.

On the other hand, the fact that full force is applied in one point (initially) implies osseous and implant overloading, not only on the tooth closest to the prematurity, but also on the rest, because of the leverage that is produced.

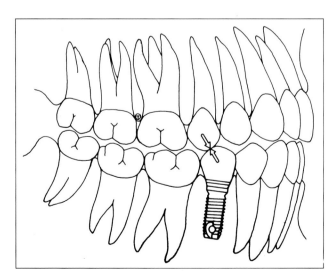

Fig. 3.6
Diagram of prematurity.

I) Interferences

These are the nonphysiological contacts that appear in the anterior and posterior teeth in lateral and protrusive excursions.

a) The nonworking interferences are very important because the mandible must pivot to avoid them, which in turn produces:

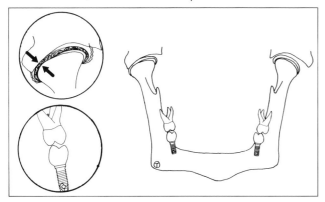

Fig. 3.7

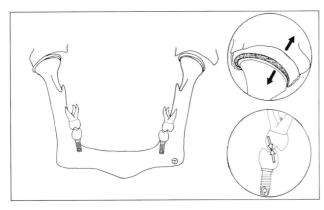

Fig. 3.8

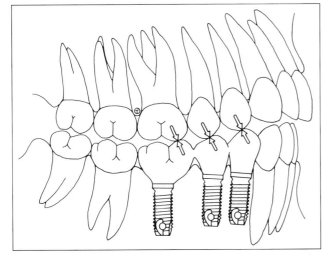

Fig. 3.9

- A compressive component on the working condyle, predisposing to arthrosis and discal pathology in their external insertions (Fig. 3.7).

- A tensional component in the nonworking condyle, which predisposes to hyperlaxitudes and meniscal displacement (Fig. 3.8).

- Overloading of the implants due to the presence of lateral forces.

b) The working interferences create large frictional surfaces in premolars and molars during lateral excursions due to the presence of multiple contacts. The lateral forces generated cause implant overloading and loss of harmony among the anatomical structures within the articular fossa.

If anterior guidance cannot be accomplished, group function should be used. This should be done following the anatomical components and obtaining contact in the first premolar, second premolar, and mesiobuccal cusp of the upper first molar (Fig. 3.9).

The presence of anterior guidance implies that posterior contacts during working movements should be eliminated (Fig. 3.10)

c) Protrusive interferences create a tensional component in both condyles and implant overloading (Fig. 3.11).

Prematurities and interferences will be more or less pathological depending on whether parafunctions are present.

During mastication, the teeth should only contact at the end (before that, a bolus exists that separates them). Contacts also occur when swallowing saliva. The duration of both functions totals approximately 10 minutes daily. If parafunctions exist, the time for both functions may increase enormously, thus causing the appearance of a traumatic factor. Unless there are remaining teeth, it will be impossible to determine the relationship between stress, parafunctions, and the patient.

The patient's occlusal restoration should not only focus on the masticatory function (as mentioned before, these occlusal contacts are not long-lasting, so they will not be of great importance) but also and particularly on parafunctions.

For this reason, avoiding prematurities and interferences is important; however, it is also important to inform patients of the dangers of clenching and grinding, which in many cases they are not aware of.

On occasion, we must protect the whole system through the use of nocturnal occlusal splints.

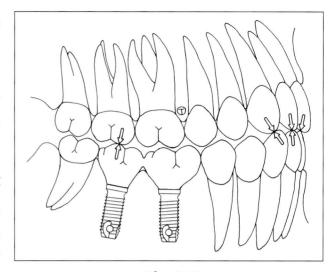

Fig. 3.10

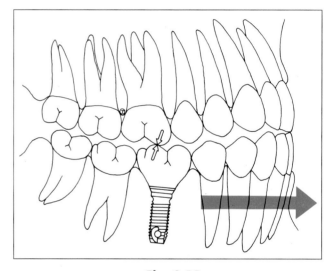

Fig. 3.11

3.2. Levers and masticatory forces

It is important to go into detail here to know how far we must extend the prosthesis and what happens should there be overloading on the anterior teeth.

The force vectors of the masticatory muscles (especially the masseter) are produced on the mesiolingual cusp of the upper first molar, making this the major loading point. Figure 3.12 shows the resultant of these force vectors of mastication and its influence on mandibular stability.

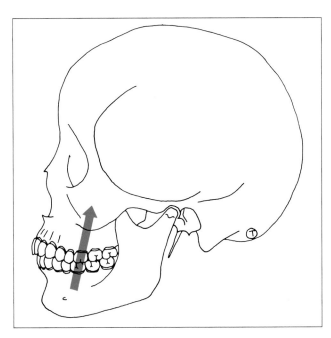

Fig. 3.12

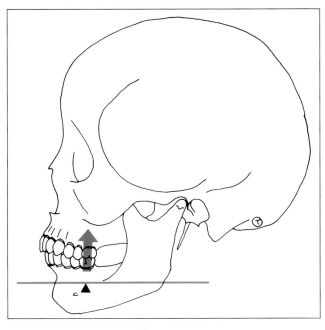

Fig. 3.14

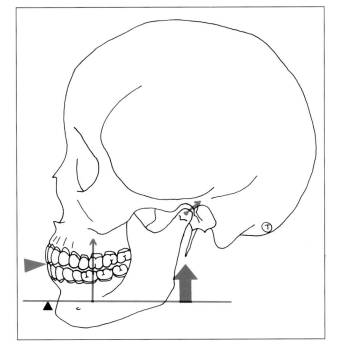

Fig. 3.13

If we can achieve contact from front to back up to the upper first molar, mandibular distalization will be avoided. Consequently, to have a stable TMJ it is important to have at least occlusion on the mesiolingual cusp of the upper first molar (Fig. 3.14).

On other hand, it must be emphasized that the anterior teeth should not contact in maximum intercuspation, because in practice it is very difficult to differentiate between physiological and excessive contacts. In maximum intercuspation, the occlusion from canine to canine should allow for a Mylar strip to be pulled with a certain resistance, yet not being fully held by the teeth. This will confirm the absence of heavy contacts there and will prevent future compressions of the posterior TMJ area.

If the first contact happens in the area of the anterior teeth, it could lead to posterior condylar displacement, producing overload capsulitis (Fig. 3.13).

3.3. Occlusion in implant-supported prostheses

A) Fixed or removable restorations with opposing natural dentition

In these cases, we recommend mutually protected occlusion, with anterior guidance and tooth-to-tooth and cusp-fossa posterior occlusion. This is also known as *organic occlusion*.

B) Fixed or removable restoration with opposing fixed or removable implant-supported prosthesis

Organic occlusion is recommended for the following reasons:

1. It is easier to produce.

2. If it is supported by mucosa and we can achieve a disocclusion as flat as possible, the tension on the implants will be minimal.

3. If a bilateral balanced occlusion is created, there will be many contact surfaces in lateral excursions, thus increasing muscular contraction force and the possibility of osseous resorption, which in turn will destabilize the mucosa-supported segment. In the case of an overdenture, this could progress into an overload of the stomatognathic system and the implants if it is not relined periodically.

Organic occlusion is easier to adjust by simply eliminating all non-anterior contacts during lateral movements. However, in the case of bilateral balanced occlusion, it could be difficult to differentiate physiological contacts from true interferences.

Even if the occlusal scheme is constructed on an articulator, we should consider that there are many factors not in harmony with anatomical and physiological realities, like the fact that the joint has soft tissues (resilience) and mandibular flexibility that on occasion produces natural positions that can't be reproduced in a rigid instrument such as the articulator.

The articulator is of great importance for prosthesis construction regardless of the type, because it brings us closer to what truly happens. Yet we believe that the final occlusal adjustments should be carried out in the mouth, because the mouth is the only articulator that provides 100% of the necessary information.

In the mouth, however, it is nearly impossible or at least very difficult to distinguish between equilibrium (physiological) contacts and interferences (non-physiological) contacts; thus, it is wiser to eliminate both (balancing or hyperbalancing contacts) so as to achieve disocclusion.

As an example to help understand this situation, imagine the muscular force needed to drag a hoop along the ground (this corresponds to canine guidance) and the force needed to drag a barrel with more surface friction the same way (this corresponds to bilateral balanced occlusion).

In 1989, Miralles, Bull, and Manns performed an electromyographic study comparing the activity of the elevator muscles (temporal and masseter) in balanced full dentures and canine-guided dentures. They found that canine guidance produces less activity in both muscles during lateral movements, which can be considered a factor in preventing parafunctional activity.

4. Organic occlusion is the most physiological scheme for the stomatognathic system and implants, but let us not forget that the patient being rehabilitated can have parafunctional problems that must not be overlooked.

5. Since there is no posterior seal in cases of implant restoration with upper overdentures, the presence of bilateral balanced occlusion does not increase retention during parafunctions, which would help initial mastication.

6. The presence of canine guidance prevents posterior tooth wear, stabilizing occlusion and avoiding parafunctions.

7. Maintainance of the neuromuscular mechanism avoids overloading of the muscular system and the appearance of trigger points.

8. In cases with only two implants supporting a lower overdenture, with adequate mucosal adjustment and seal, it is advisable to use bilaterally balanced occlusion. This will improve prosthesis stability and avoid implant overload.

C) Fixed or removable implant-supported restoration with opposing removable full denture without implants

This is the case in which we advocate bilaterally balanced occlusion. Here it is perfectly logical.

In conventional full dentures (without implants), teeth are arranged in bilateral balance when the patient is not chewing, during parafunctions and with teeth clenching in different positions. Forces are transmitted evenly, resulting in a more stable prosthesis with increased adhesion and fit, which will benefit patient food mastication.

We should not forget that, while eating, the food bolus separates occlusal surfaces, consequently neutralizing balance. However, the adhesion that was previously produced through bilateral balanced occlusion greatly facilitates chewing without denture displacement, through a "vacuum-type" effect.

We support bilateral balanced occlusion because we look for increased full-denture stability in patients without implants.

D) Partial-prosthesis occlusion

In cases with cantilevers, the resilience of the neighboring natural dentition and of the TMJ should be taken into consideration.

The recommended occlusion in these cases is adjusted for forced biting. In this way, resilience will be introduced into the occlusal adjustment, and in this forced position we omit the contacts. The prosthesis should only contact in a position of forced closure.

As always, all interferences and prematurities should be eliminated with care, leaving only pointlike occlusion.

E) Single-implant occlusion

Single implants should be free of any occlusal overload and function. The lingual surface of the anterior teeth should be constructed as flat as possible, so if opposing tooth extrusion leads to occlusal contact there will not be contacts in lateral movements.

Single implants in the posterior area should be limited to premolars, reducing their surface area so that they just fulfill esthetics and space maintenance.

At this time we do not advocate the use of single implants for molars. The only solution here is the placement of two implants in the place of the mesial and distal roots to serve as support for a molar.

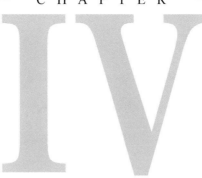

OCCLUSAL ADJUSTMENT IN IMPLANT-SUPPORTED PROSTHESES

4.1 General aspects

This consists of modifying tooth anatomy to obtain a good occlusion.

The objectives are the following:

— To have centric relation and maximum intercuspation coincide.

— To create better anterior guidance.

— To position cusps.

— To deepen fossae.

— To change inclines.

— To locate the exit paths.

— To build in vertical-dimension holding contacts to avoid implant overloading.

— To eliminate prematurities and interferences.

Occlusal adjustment must be performed in the upper and lower arch jointly, at the same time, and on both sides.

All of the following adjustments refer to implant-supported prostheses, either when checking a case prior to laboratory work, or once it is placed in the mouth, or in finished cases where it is decided to readjust the occlusion. They can also be used in natural dentition.

4.2. Technique

There are many different occlusal-adjustment technique philosophies; however, they all lead to a common goal, explained previously.

We will make a compendium of those techniques taught to us by our teachers (López Alvarez, Stuart, del Río, Casado, Cordoba, Martínez Ross, Curnutte, Solnit, Guichet, López Viejo, Mariano Sanz, López López, López Lozano, etc) and try to summarize their most important ideas in a logical and simple manner.

First, the case is mounted on an articulator with a face bow related to the orbital point and the hinge axis, to get a "general idea" of the treatment the patient needs.

We deliberately used the term "general idea," as mentioned before, because the final adjustment will be carried out directly in the mouth. However, we should look for information on prematurities and interferences, and whether canine or anterior guidance is feasible. In our opinion, and considering that articulators are not perfect since they do not simulate soft tissues, we do not feel it is necessary to complicate initial phases with previous registrations (orthopanography) but we must register the patient's condylar inclination.

The information we wish to obtain can be determined through the use of a semiadjustable articulator (Dentatus, Denar Mark II, etc). It is very important, once we have analyzed the case, to know where we want to start and determine our objective. We believe that it is fundamental to have centric relation and maximum intercuspation coincide, eliminating all prematurities. We try to avoid cusp-tip contact with the floor of the fossa, allowing only point-like contacts with the internal fossa walls, so as to avoid large contact surfaces that can lead to implant overloading.

Once we have achieved anterior coupling, we eliminate the interferences (Fig. 4.1). In some cases, we will need more than one appointment to obtain this.

A) Eliminating prematurities

To mark tooth contacts, we use double-colored thin articulating paper or black marking ribbon and we have the patient close from centric relation (CR) to maximum intercuspation (MI) several times.

1) Mandible

To adjust the lower occlusion, we should remember that in normal occlusion (Class I) the lower teeth (premolars and molars) are

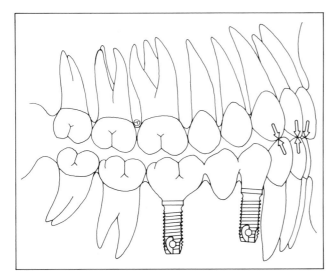

Fig. 4.1

ahead of the upper.

So we can observe that when occlusion occurs, the distal lower inclines and the mesial upper inclines contact in condylar centric relation.

To adjust, we should follow these steps:

1.I   Cusp distal inclines

Eliminate the most distal part (DI) and preserve the most mesial contact point (M) (Fig. 4.2).

1.II   Active-cusp outer inclines

Eliminate the whole surface except the zone next to the cusp tip (the highest part) (Fig. 4.3).

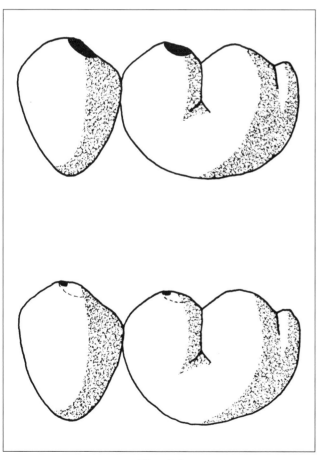

Fig. 4.2

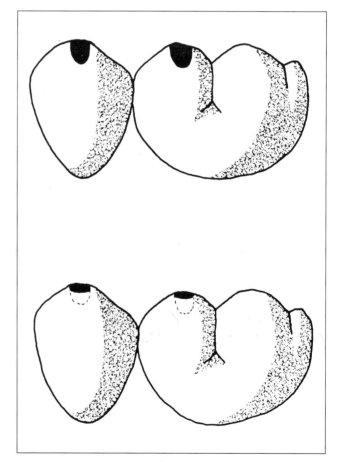

Fig. 4.3

1.III Inner inclines

Eliminate the most distal area (DI), except for the most mesial and medial contact point (anterior and towards the center of the fossa) (Fig. 4.4).

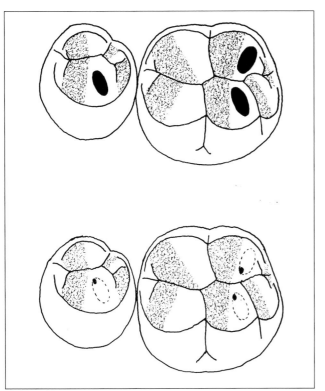

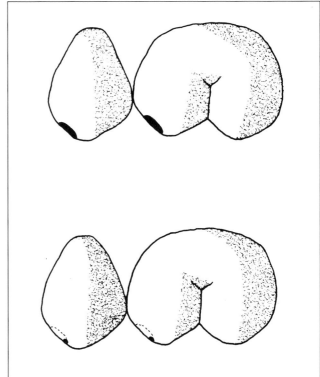

Fig. 4.4   **Fig. 4.5**

2) Maxilla

In the upper arch we always adjust opposite of the lower arch.

2.I Mesial cusp inclines

Eliminate the most mesial part and leave the most distal contact point.

2.II Active-cusp outer inclines

Eliminate the whole surface, except for the area nearest to the active cusp tip (the lowest part) (Fig. 4.6).

2.III Inner inclines

Eliminate the most mesial and leave the most distal and medial contact point (Fig. 4.7).

B) Deepening fossae: maxilla and mandible

If the cusp contacts the floor of the fossa, it will create a large contact surface, which we always try to avoid. There are two possibilities:

a)   Spare the lateral cusp marks while eliminating the intermediate zone, which will cause loss of active material for chewing and will decrease efficiency (Fig. 4.8).

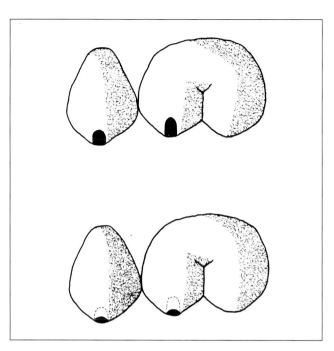

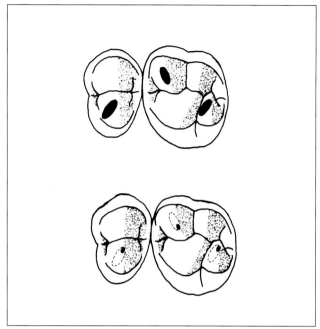

Fig. 4.6   **Fig. 4.7**

b) Deepen the fossa while preserving its lateral aspects, which will permit preservation of the cusp surface (Fig. 4.9).

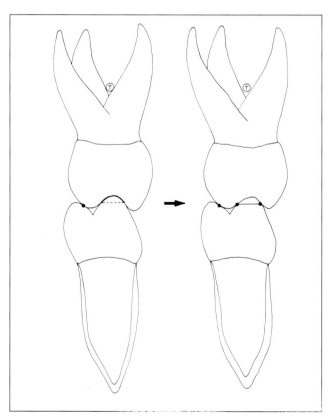

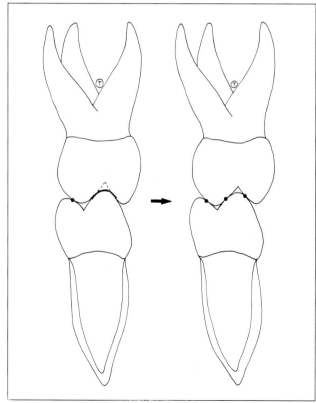

Fig. 4.8   **Fig. 4.9**

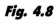

The best solution is the second one, because it will preserve active cusp anatomy and masticatory activity. Occlusal maintenance contacts will still be present.

The large surface marking that appears on the cusp tip after deepening the opposing fossa will be reduced simply to two contact points.

It should be emphasized that the thinnest possible black double-colored marking ribbon should be used while eliminating prematurities and deepening fossa, placing it in the mouth and having the patient close from centric relation to maximum intercuspation.

At the end of this phase of adjustment a great number of black contact points, not surfaces, will appear on the occlusal surfaces.

The presence or absence of excessive contact in the anterior teeth must be checked during closure. It should be done with very thin ribbon, noting slight resistance while pulling it from the teeth.

The next step is to verify anterior guidance.

C) Anterior guidance

The anterior guidance should be as flat as possible to avoid overload in the anterior teeth in lateral excursion (on the canines and anterior teeth) and in protrusion (the contact of the mesial incline of the first lower premolar on the distal incline of the upper canine, as well as centrals, laterals, and canines between them).

As the desired occlusal scheme was detailed previously, we shall merely emphasize that we must avoid producing TMJ tension and any contact in the posterior when the guidance is in function, because these would constitute interferences. This is always checked with red marking ribbon, allowing for fine surfaces of anterior disocclusion.

D) Eliminating interferences

For this, we must again use red ribbon and have the patient go through working, nonworking, and protrusive movements.

The next step is to place black ribbon and have the patient close to maximum intercuspation (centric relation coincides at this time with maximum intercuspation). All surfaces or points that appear which are not black must be eliminated (except black on red); in other words, eliminate all red marking except the guide marks of anterior disocclusion. When these red markings coincide with shallow or nonexistent disocclusion, it is convenient to eliminate them following the corresponding direction, depending if they are working, nonworking, or protrusive movements (see chapter III).

The importance of inducing lateral movements to detect if Bennett movement is present must not be forgotten.

4.3. Conclusions

Occlusal adjustment is necessary in any kind of fixed or removable restoration supported by implants.

If we have opposing natural dentition, we must be sure that the introduction of new cusps in the rehabilitation does not create occlusal problems in the opposing dentition. If this happens, we should adjust the natural dentition without hesitation.

If the opposing dentition is a full denture that is not implant-supported, we can bypass the techniques involving physiological interferences because we are dealing with a bilateral balanced occlusion; however, we must take care in eliminating prematurities.

When adjusting the occlusion on partial prostheses, the contacts created must occur during forced biting and at the same time as the rest, avoiding the introduction of new prematurities or interferences. The opposing natural dentition must also be checked.

Occlusion in single implants was explained in chapter III.

Because of possible TMJ and occlusal instability, periodic occlusal checkups (every 3 to 6 months) are strongly recommended.

Occlusal problems will cause bone resorption at the implant site. On occasion, this is why screws loosen, though sometimes this is related to the lack of passive fit of the prosthesis over the abutments.

4.4 Occlusal splints

If it becomes necessary to protect the occlusion of the stomatognathic system from parafunctions and overloads, acrylic-resin nocturnal occlusal splints are indicated. In these cases we search for canine guidance in lateral excursions, disoccluding anterior guidance in protrusions, and posterior fossa wall contacts against the opposing active cusp tips that will serve as the deepest part of the corresponding fossa.

Guidance should be as flat as possible; if the distribution of occlusal leverages permits it (minimum occlusal contacts up to the first molar), an upper occlusal splint is employed. If an upper splint is not feasible, a lower splint is used.

The posterior occlusal zone must be absolutely flat and the anterior concave, without any kind of tooth print, so as to allow freedom of movement in maximum intercuspation and laterally. It must relax the TMJ muscle complex, guiding the mandible to centric relation without any impediments. The presence of minimal contacts and the absence of interferences and prematurities reduces muscular forces during parafunctions (bruxism).

Occlusal adjustment will be undertaken considering the contact markings with their corresponding fossae and upper inner inclines, eliminating the rest that do not correspond to the lower active cusps (see fossae adjustment and upper inner inclines). This should be checked periodically. If this should change with the appearance of new prematurities or interferences, it indicates that mandibular position is changing, so special attention must be given to the patient's new occlusion if a occlusal splint is not being used. The implant-supported prosthesis and the natural teeth (should they be present) must be readjusted.

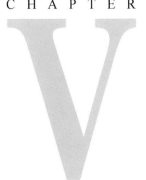

CHAPTER

V

ANTERIOR GROUP
DIFFICULTIES

The use of implants to restore a single tooth is one the most important achievements of dentistry in the last few years.

Before this, the loss of an upper central incisor would probably have been solved with a fixed prosthesis from canine to canine, as well as endodontic treatment of at least the laterals and in many cases of the entire anterior segment. Teeth had to be reinforced with cast posts, and besides tooth-preparation difficulties, we faced two other problems: the gingiva and esthetics.

Today, with state-of-art prosthodontic accessories such as the CeraOne abutment, we can achieve perfect esthetics, since we do not have to use metal. Instead, we now have a prefabricated alumina base, onto which we place porcelain, that offers perfect shoulder adjustment. To use this accessory subgingivally, the implant must be positioned perfectly in the alveolar ridge, so the crown emerges from the gingiva centrally positioned in relation to the adjacent natural teeth.

This does not always happen, so on occasion we can still use the standard transepithelial cylindrical abutment, which will produce acceptable esthetics. If the implant's inclination is to the buccal, angulated abutments can be used.

When dealing with difficulties in the anterior teeth, we will have four options:

a) Well-positioned implants with favorable esthetics: use CeraOne or tapered abutments.

b) Poorly positioned implants with unfavorable esthetics due to lingualization or high emergence: use standard abutments.

c) Poorly positioned implants with unfavorable esthetics due to buccalization: use angulated abutments.

d) Well-positioned implants with unfavorable esthetics because of high smile line showing elongated teeth, also related to excessive interarch distance: use standard or tapered abutments.

Next we will detail each of these options:

5.1 CeraOne System

A) Case 1. Patient with missing upper central incisor: technique, clinical, and laboratory procedures are described.

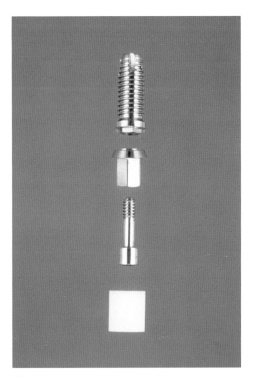

Fig. 5.1

Implant, CeraOne abutment, screw, and alumina coping (cap).

Fig. 5.2

Surgical phase with the implant positioned adequately, centered on the alveolar ridge (courtesy of Dr. Ramón Martínez).

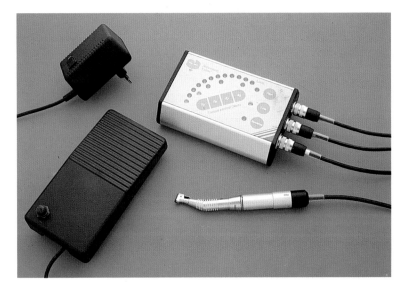

Fig. 5.3

Torque-control driver used to affix the holding screw of the CeraOne to the implant with a force of 32 Ncm, thus preventing the screw from loosening. Should we need to change it later, this machine can be used again counterclockwise with a force of 45 Ncm. It can also apply forces of 10 N to fix the prosthesis to the implant in the mouth.

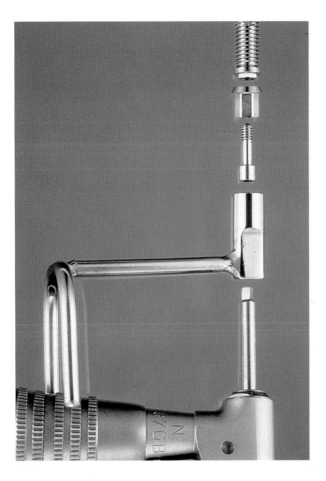

Fig. 5.4

Antirotational accessory to avoid implant tensions.

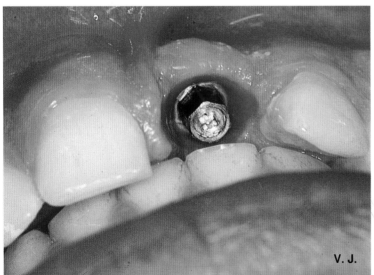

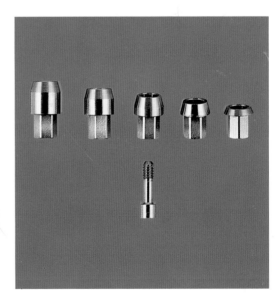

V. J.

Figs. 5.5 and 5.6

CeraOne abutment screwed to the implant. Notice its hexagonal base that avoids crown rotation in the mouth, as well as its subgingival shoulder. Various abutment lengths are available to improve esthetics by positioning the shoulder more subgingivally. The screw is made of gold so it attains better resistance. Notice that the surrounding gingiva has healed, indicating that at least 15 to 20 days have elapsed since abutment placement.

V

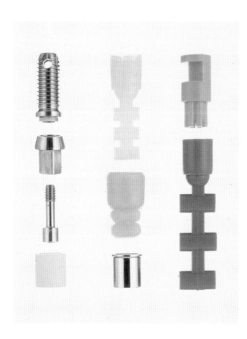

Fig. 5.7

CeraOne abutment accessories. Starting on the left from top to bottom is the implant, CeraOne cylinder, screw that holds both together, and alumina coping (on top of which the porcelain crown is constructed in the laboratory).

In the center from top to bottom, are two accessories for provisionals; the white one corresponds to upper laterals and lower incisors, and the yellow one corresponds to upper centrals and premolars, with a wider width to better imitate the tooth emergence from the gingiva. Under them there is usually a metal coping; a burnout castable coping (not pictured) is also available for posterior cases. On the right is the yellow-colored cylinder replica that is an exact copy of the hexagonal base and reproduces the shoulder precisely.

We will obtain an exact duplicate of the CeraOne in the mouth when we place it in the impression accessory (blue transfer coping). The transfer coping (right side of picture) fits precisely on the hexagonal base of the abutment, and it can be reduced to desired height.

Since the alumina coping fits with precision to the hexagonal base and the abutment shoulder, this will contribute to prosthesis adjustment and lack of rotation when placed in the mouth. Metal is not used to construct the crown so as to enhance esthetics.

Fig. 5.8

Once the transfer coping blue has been placed in the mouth and shortened, we can proceed to take the impression (always use a syringe). Any fluid silicone may be used to reproduce gingival anatomy, but it must be strong enough to avoid tearing when the impression tray is removed from the mouth. In the picture, the transfer coping is shown placed in the tray once the impression has been taken. It is important to check that no excess material has flowed into the hexagonal base; should this occur, it would indicate that the adjustment in the mouth was faulty, and we would have to repeat the procedure.

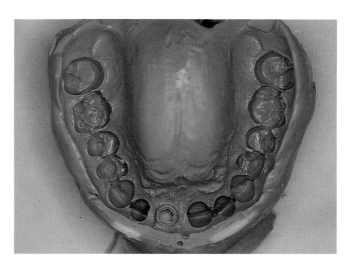

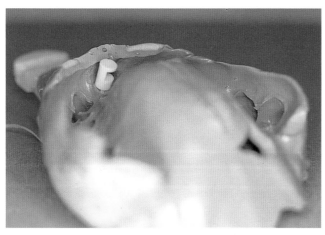

Fig. 5.9

We proceed to position the CeraOne replica (positive) into the impression (negative) to exactly duplicate on the cast what occurs in the mouth.

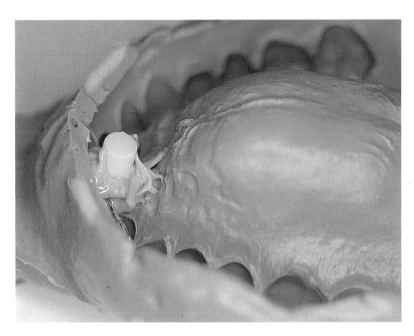

Fig. 5.10

It is convenient to construct a soft tissue model using polysulfides to prevent the silicone from sticking and to have a removable gingival model. The rest of the cast is poured afterwards.

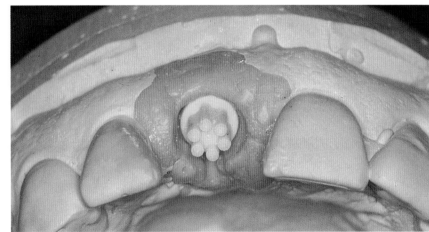

Fig. 5.11

The cast has been made and the gingiva appears in pink. The soft tissue can be removed and fitted back. The picture also shows the hexagonal base with a circumferential flat shoulder.

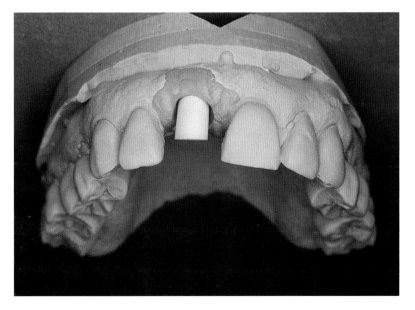

Fig. 5.12

The alumina coping is placed over the replica. By removing the gingiva, we can check the shoulder fit. Anterior view.

V

Fig. 5.13

Lingual view of the alumina coping. Notice its concave shape to achieve better anatomy. Through the small buccal window we can see the perfect adjustment.

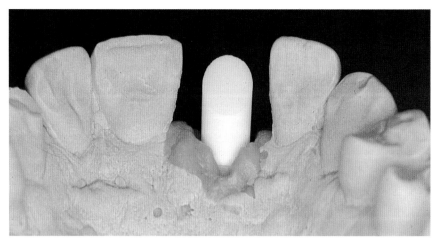

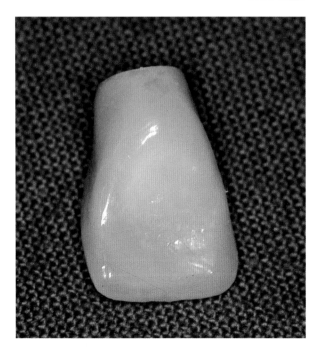

Fig. 5.14

The crown has been completed in the laboratory by placing dentin and enamel. From this upper view we can see that the shoulder of the alumina coping is absolutely clean. This will couple to the Cera-One abutment shoulder in the mouth. This is achieved by precise prefabrication.

Fig. 5.15

Lingual view of the finished crown. Notice the incisal translucency and yellow interproximal stains, which are also present in the patient's mouth.

It is important to know that in these cases the crown is cemented and that is why there is no entry orifice for the screw.

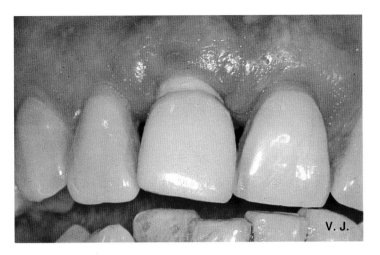

Fig. 5.16

During the healing phase, an adjusted temporary acrylic-resin tooth is placed on the single provisional accessory. Its construction is very simple, using a tooth previsously made in the laboratory and rebasing it in the mouth by introducing temporary acrylic into the crown and adjusting it afterwards. A full-denture tooth can be used by hollowing it out and rebasing it with acrylic resin for a good fit over the provisional abutment. It should be relieved for better gingival healing.

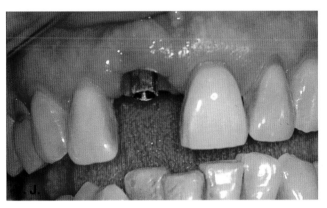
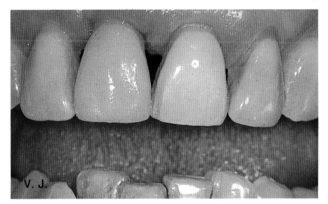

Figs. 5.17 and 5.18

Case before and after: notice the good esthetic result. The patient had some teeth with stains impossible to remove, and we wanted to provide treatment with complementary esthetics.

We are dealing with the upper anterior area that usually has great bone quantity, permitting the use of long implants.

Care should be taken, as we will see in the next case, to ensure at least 1 or 2 mm separation between apexes to avoid causing pathology in adjacent teeth. Any kind of zinc phosphate cement may be used. Once it sets, the excess is easily removed. Cement is brushed on the external aspect of the hexagonal base and the crown placed over it.

B) Case 2. Missing upper lateral incisor. Patient has periodontal involvement, with a composite splint of the two central incisors. The patient previously had orthodontic treatment, which produced apical resorption of the anterior teeth. The missing upper lateral was to be replaced through prosthodontics.

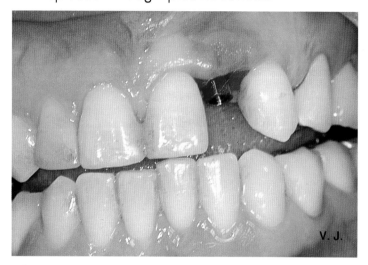

Fig. 5.19

CeraOne abutment in the mouth; observe the splinting of the two upper central incisors.

Fig. 5.20

Occlusal view of the CeraOne abutment.

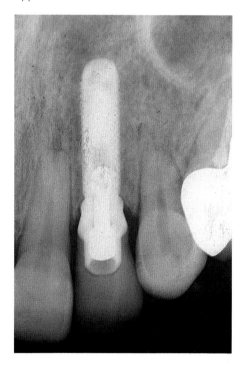

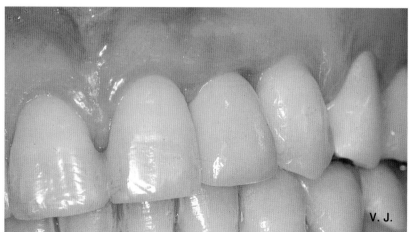

Fig. 5.21

The radiograph shows the good implant length, adjacent apical resorption, and perfect prosthesis fit.

Fig. 5.22

Completed case. Even though we are dealing with a lateral, if we follow the technique described previously, good tooth emergence from the gingiva can be obtained. The diameter should be a bit smaller than that of the central incisors.

C) Case 3. Missing upper lateral incisor and lacerated gingiva: 1-year follow-up.

When we began to construct the prosthesis, we noticed that the gingiva was somewhat lacerated. Nevertheless, we decided to finish it, cement it, and recall the patient every 3 months. Emphasis was placed on achieving a good proximal contact, and we informed the patient about the importance of oral hygiene.

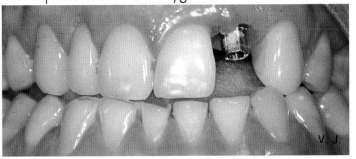

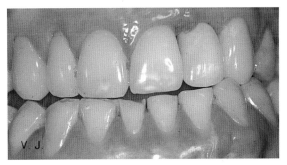

Fig. 5.23

Observe the poor occlusion, as well as the wear facets indicating the presence of bruxism. The patient wore a nocturnal occlusal splint.

Fig. 5.24

Finished case presenting inflammation of the mesial aspect, as well as loss of free gingiva.

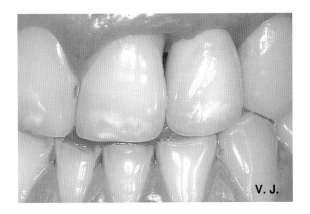

Fig. 5.25

Three months later, the gingiva is no longer inflamed and is beginning to regenerate. Emphasis must be placed on obtaining interproximal contact and a perfect fit of the crown to its base.

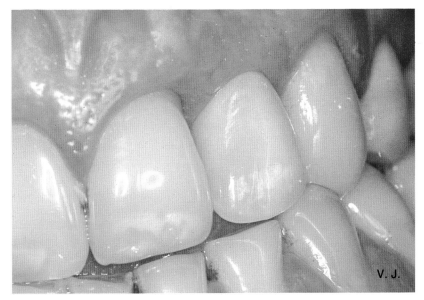

Fig. 5.26

The gingiva has regenerated and the goal has been accomplished. We have done our job (good contact point and good alumina coping adjustment to the CeraOne shoulder) and nature has taken care of the rest.

D) Case 4. Tooth repositioning without interdental papilla: two solutions.

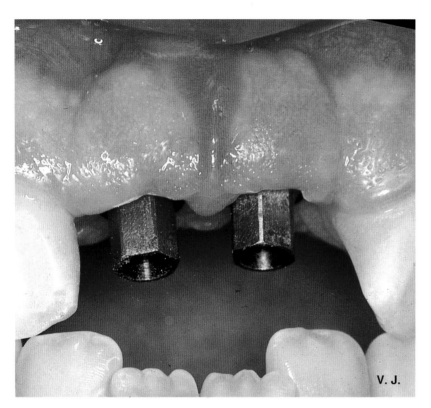

Fig. 5. 27

The patient presents this situation before construction of the prosthesis of the two upper central incisors. We chose to build two independent crowns with the CeraOne system.

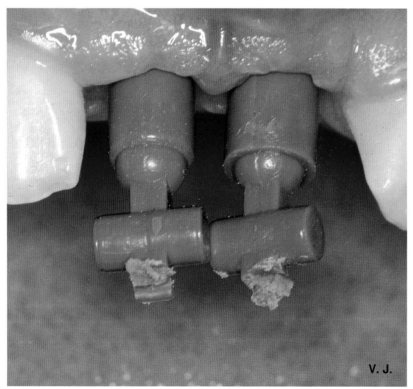

Fig. 5.28

Try-in of transfer copings that have been shortened so that they do not interfere with the impression, yet are retentive enough to be picked up by the impression tray once the silicone has hardened. There is no need for a customized tray and the silicone impression can be done in one appointment.

V

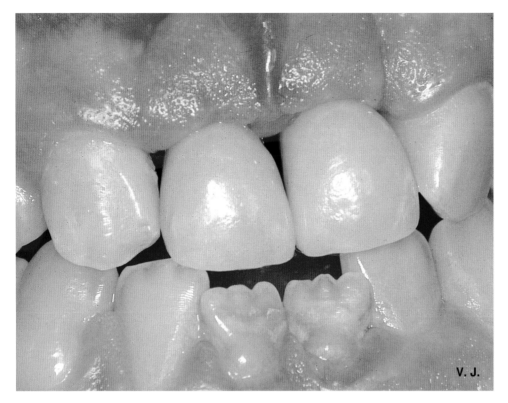

V. J.

Figs. 5.29 and 5.30

The patient was offered two solutions. In the picture at the top, the papillae are free so as to make patient hygiene easier.

In the picture at the bottom, the papillae space was closed and esthetics are somewhat improved. The patient chose the second option, despite our recommendation.

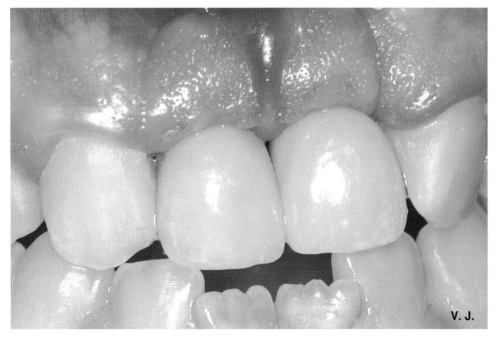

V. J.

E) Case 5. Missing upper canines: occlusal solution.

In this case we must replace the two missing upper canines. The laterals that appear in the picture aren't really laterals but canines that could not be repositioned and were treated with esthetic veneers by Dr. José María Botella. Anterior guidance will be developed on these teeth and the centrals.

The canines that lack occlusal function will only serve for esthetics. (Courtesy of Dr. Juan Canut.)

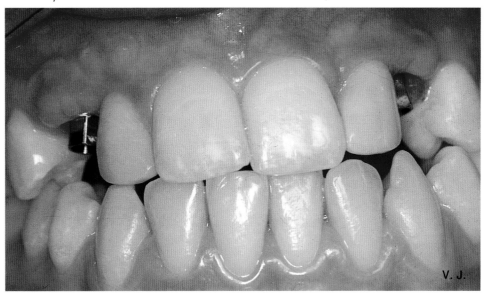

Figs. 5.31 and 5.32

Before and after. Notice that the occlusion in the canine replacements has been relieved (see Fig. 12.23).

F) **Case 6.** Lower incisor difficulties. In these cases, due to implant width, it is very difficult to solve these problems at the gingival margin. They may be solved in the near future with new prosthetic accessories and narrower implants. Basically, the difficulty lies in the alumina coping width, on top of which dentin must be placed, making if difficult to obtain a more slender tooth.

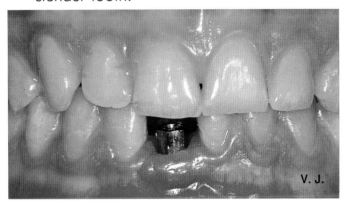
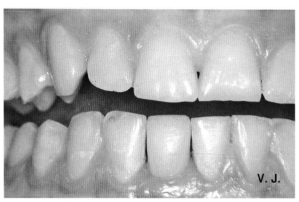

Figs. 5.33 and 5.34

Before and after. Observe that the width at the gingival margin is slightly greater than that of the neighboring natural incisors.

G) **Case 7.** Immediate implants. A 20-year-old patient presented with a traumatic fracture of the left upper central incisor. Since it could not be saved, it was extracted and an implant was placed immediately.

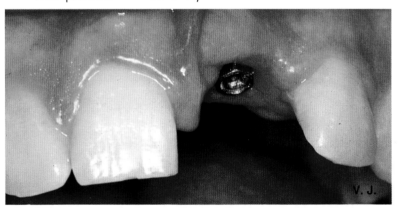

Figs. 5.35 and 5.36

Before and after.

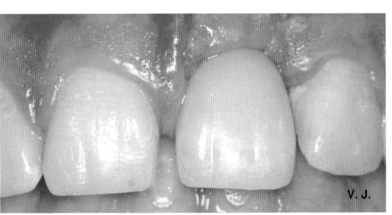

H) Case 8. Implants and reimplantation.

This probably is the case that has taken us the longest to solve.

In 1980 the patient experienced traumatic avulsion of the upper right central incisor. The patient came to the office with the tooth in hand 24 hours later. After endodontics, the tooth was reimplanted and splinted with composite resin. Calcium hydroxide was placed previously in the alveolus.

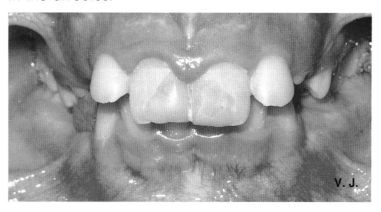

Fig. 5.37

Tooth reimplanted and splinted with composite resin. Observe the large overbite. The patient was referred to an orthodontist, who began studying the case.

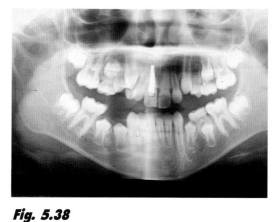

Fig. 5.38

This panoramic radiograph corresponds to the study prior to treatment (courtesy of Dr. Javier Alvarez Carlón). Subsequent radiograph controls demonstrated the existence of a large radicular resorption.

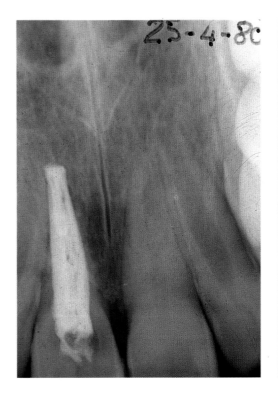
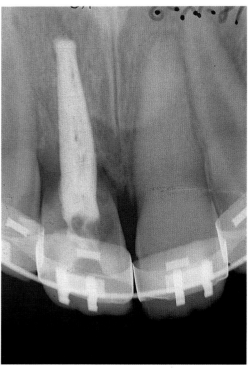

Figs. 5.39 and 5.40

Notice the large resorption that occurred in 12 months (courtesy of Dr. Pedro Badanelli).

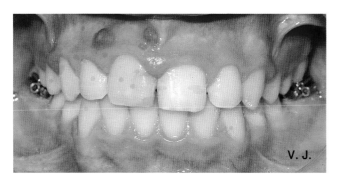
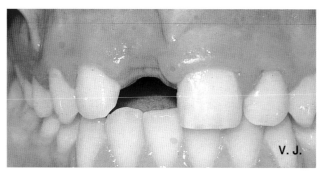

Figs. 5.41 and 5.42

Years later, a fistula showed up in the soft tissues. It was decided to have the tooth extracted (courtesy of Dr. Alvarez Carlón). Compare the great occlusal difference at the beginning of treatment with the present.

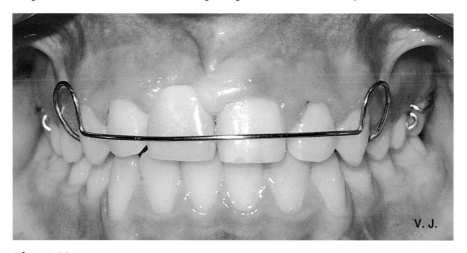

Fig. 5.43

During the remainder of the orthodontic treatment, a provisional was placed until we could finish the case.

The total length of treatment, from the avulsion to the CeraOne with a final porcelain crown, was approximately 10 years.

This is the nice thing about dentistry: "being able to work as a team knowing the merit belongs to everyone and to no one."

Fig 5.44

The case is finished and the right central incisor was replaced by an implant-supported porcelain crown. Should the gingiva not respond in the near future, a small gingivectomy will have to performed.

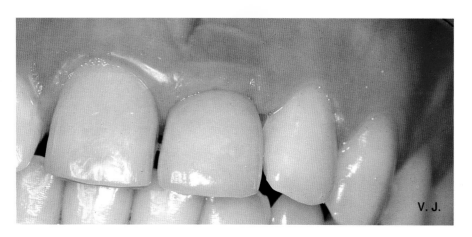

V

5.2 Standard cylindrical transepithelial abutments

They are indicated in these cases:

- The implants are placed lingually.
  There is considerable distance between the implant and the opposing tooth or arch.
- Esthetics are not a major factor, and the patient does not show any gingiva.
- There is great risk of porcelain fracture due to parafunctions. Metal occlusal surfaces are feasible with these abutments.
- Short implant length is necessary; here splinting will improve prognosis.

A) Case 1. System, clinical, and laboratory description in two upper central incisors.

This case corresponds to a patient that did not show the abutment while smiling, due to high gingival line. The patient was under periodontal treatment for bone loss. This is a description of all phases involved in the construction of the prosthesis.

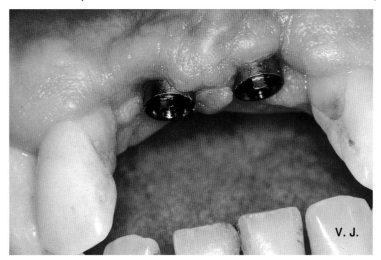

V. J.

Fig. 5.45

This is the case once the standard abutments were placed. They are cylindrical and fit into the implant through an internal hexagon that anchors it, thus avoiding rotation, and a screw that keeps it in place.

There are several sizes and the one selected must not protrude much above the gingiva. The distance to the gingiva plus the distance to the opposing tooth must also be considered. This is because the gold cylinder in the prosthesis that fits on the abutment will need a minimum distance of 6 mm.

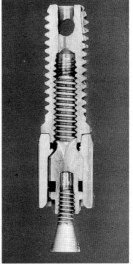

Fig. 5.46

Standard abutment connected to the implant.

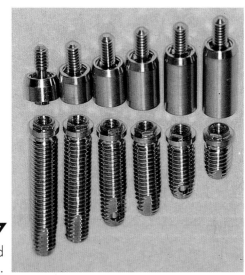

Fig. 5.47

Different models of standard abutments and implants.

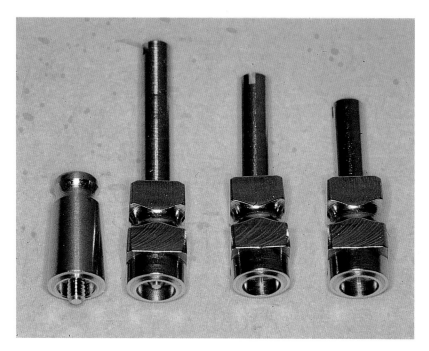

Fig. 5.48

Different accessories for abutment impression-taking. Because there are different screw sizes, we must select one with adequate height to fit through the window of the customized tray, which was previously prepared in the laboratory, facilitating the impression procedures (see Laboratory Procedures, chapter XII).

Fig. 5.49

Impression copings placed on the standard abutments. Afterward they were splinted with Duralay acrylic resin.

We take the impression with silicone, placing the analogs in position and pouring the impression.

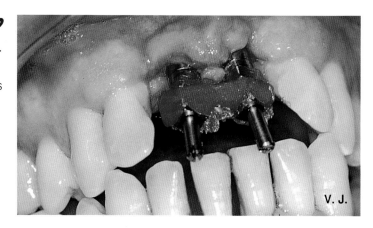

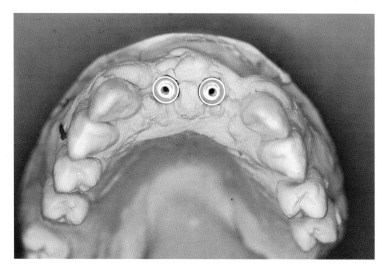

Fig. 5.50

Cast model with analogs. They have the same shape as those in the mouth. In this case, they are slightly lingualized with respect to neighboring teeth.

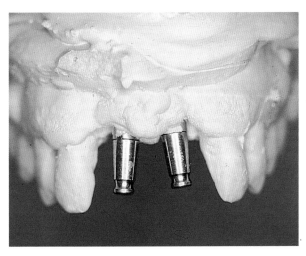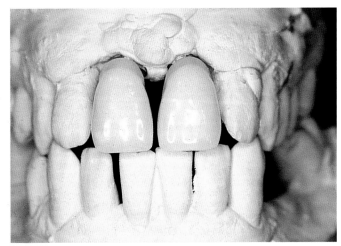

Figs. 5.51 and 5.52

Hydrocolloid transfer copings or laboratory waxup screws are placed once we have selected their length, and standard full-denture teeth are tried in to verify the screw exit in relation to esthetics.

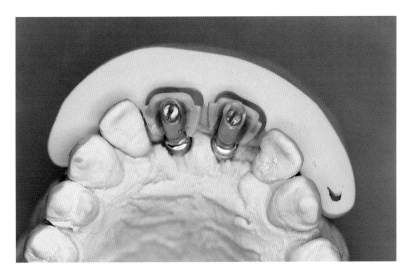

Fig. 5.53

The gold cylinder is affixed with the selected screw. Part of the complex is covered with a piece of plastic (obtained from a pen refill). This will be the future chimney.

Afterward, a prefabricated plastic wax structure is placed in relation to the silicone index obtained from the design in the previous picture to verify whether there is space enough for the porcelain.

Fig. 5.54

The space is filled with wax until an even structure is formed; we also must consider the occlusion and the interproximal contact points.

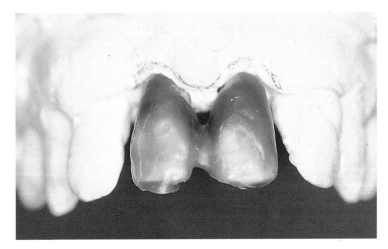

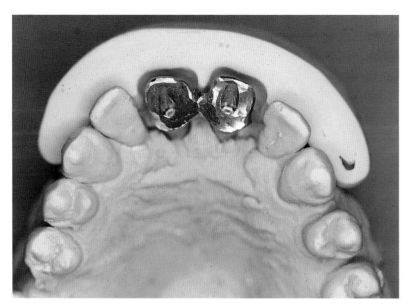

Fig. 5.55

Once cast, it is checked again to evaluate whether there is enough space for the porcelain.

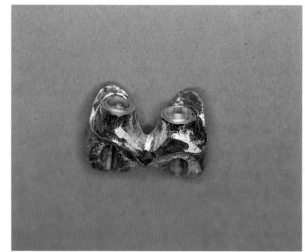

Fig. 5.56

Observe how the gold cylinder is included in the cast and a small anterior cuff has been carefully developed to buccalize the crown and improve esthetics.

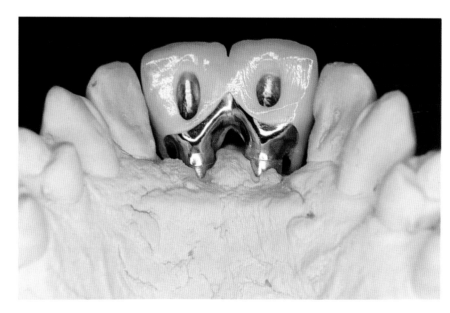

Fig. 5.57

Lingual view, where we can see the entry hole for the screw that will hold the prosthesis to the abutment. Both crowns are splinted, but they allow for good hygiene.

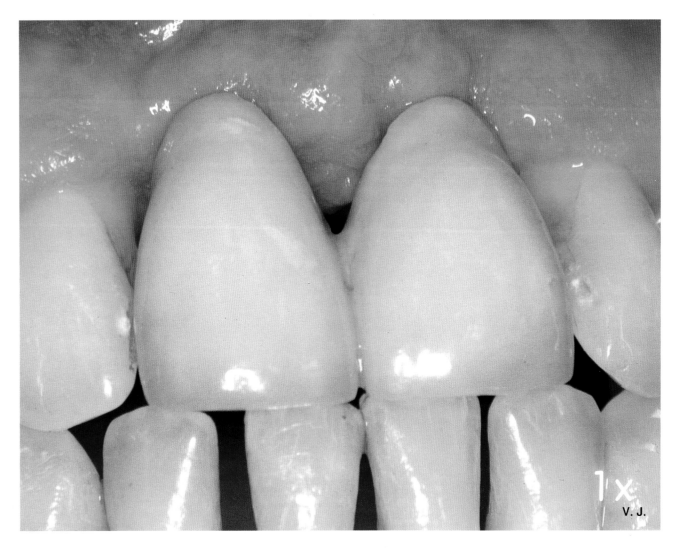

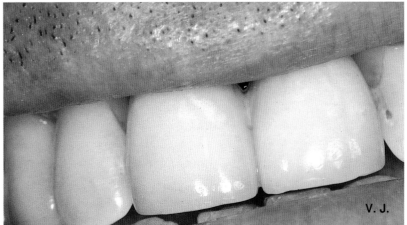

Figs. 5.58 and 5.59

The case finished and installed, showing the patient's smile line where gingiva cannot be seen. Observe that it will be easy to use the interproximal brush. The anterior cuff must be cleaned with Superfloss or water spray.

5.3 Angulated abutments

A) Case 1. Description of the system, clinical, and laboratory procedure in an upper and lower restoration, emphasizing the anterior teeth.

This patient needed a full-mouth restoration. We are going to focus only on the anterior area, where we needed to change the standard abutments because the angulation forced us to exit the screws through the buccal aspect of the crown.

We changed the standard abutments for angulated ones to obtain an inclination of 30°, compatible with good esthetics.

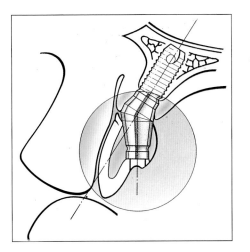

Fig. 5.60

Drawing of the angulated abutment.

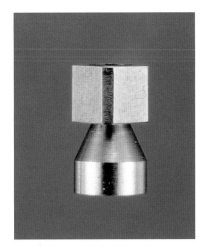

Fig. 5.61

Transfer coping for angulated abutment impressions.

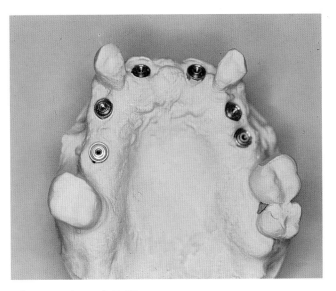
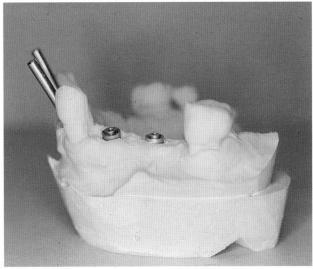

Figs. 5.62 and 5.63

Cast model of the case, in which all the abutments are standard. The direction of the screw pins in the anterior can be seen toward the buccal.

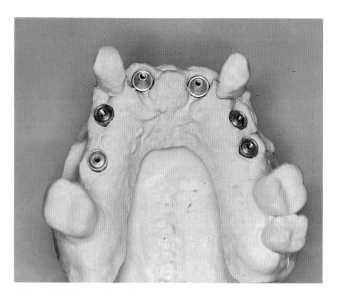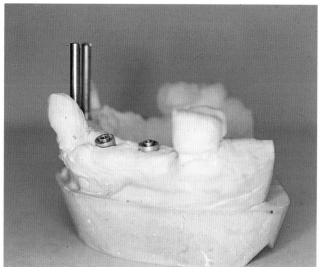

Figs. 5.64 and 5.65

New cast model, after changing the anterior abutments for angulated ones and taking a new impression. Observe that the direction of the screw pins has now changed toward the lingual.

Figs. 5.66 and 5.67

Case before and after. Notice how the central and lateral incisors are splinted over the two implants with angulated abutments, positioned at the same level as the laterals (see section 5.5, case 2).

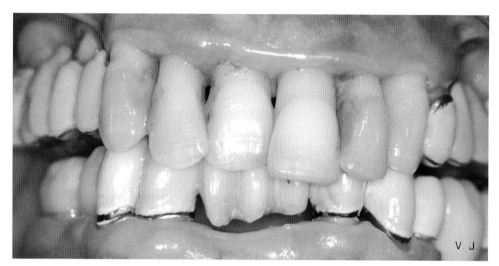

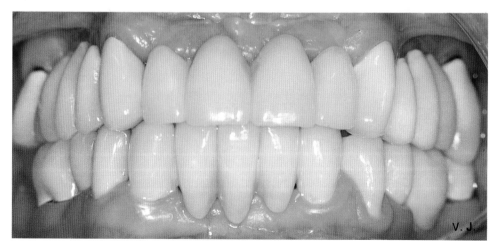

V

5.4 Unfavorable esthetics related to excessive tooth length

Although the implants might be well-placed in these cases, the problem lies in the excessive length the teeth need to achieve contact with the opposing dentition and establish good anterior guidance, which is essential.

If we add to this circumstance the fact that the patient shows a large surface while smiling, we find that the only solution is to employ hard acrylic-resin artificial gingiva, which does not need retentive attachments. This way we can have access to the interproximal space, once removed, for good oral hygiene.

Here we accomplish three objectives:
- Decreased tooth length.
- Allowance for good hygiene.
- Provision for lip support, a common problem facing fixed upper restorations.

In its construction, we must consider interproximal gingival space design to allow for sufficient parallelism that will permit its installment in an anteroposterior direction. This must be verified with a surveyor.

A) Case 1. Esthetic problem.

Initially, the patient had chosen an upper overdenture, but later preferred a fixed solution.

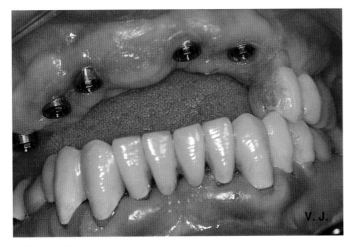

Fig. 5.68

Five standard abutments in the upper arch.

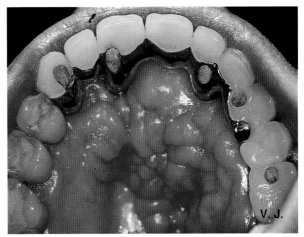

Fig. 5.69

Occlusal view of the finished case in the mouth.

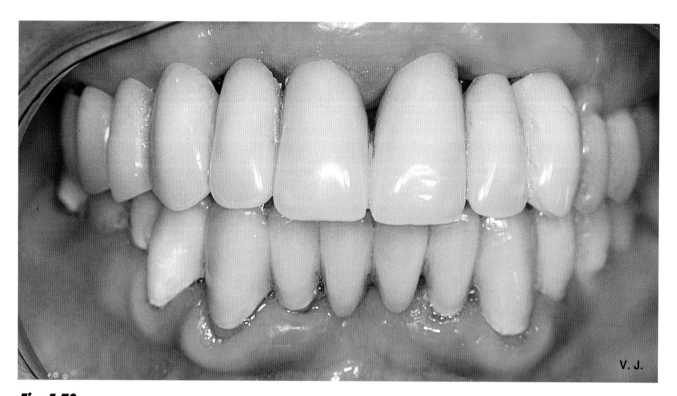

Fig. 5.70

Anterior view. Excessively long teeth contributed to disproportionate esthetics.

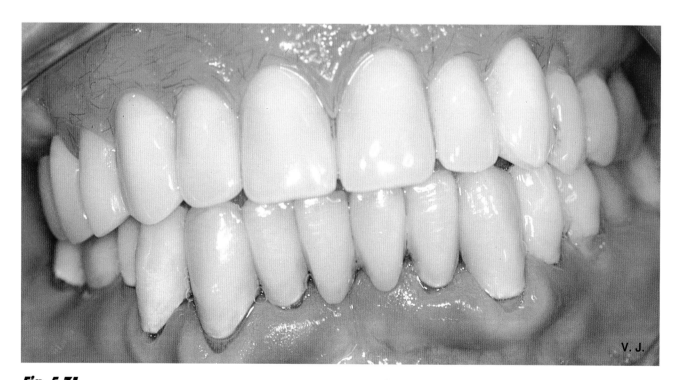

Fig. 5.71

Hard acrylic-resin artificial gingiva is placed, made with small veins in an orange-peel-type imitation of the gingiva.

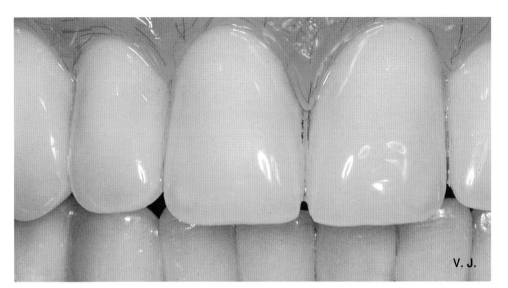

Fig. 5.72

Close-up of the anterior teeth.

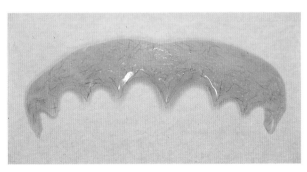

Fig. 5.73

Buccal aspect of the rigid artificial gingiva. We usually make three to four gingivae in case of fracture or loss.

Soft material is not recommended, because long-term results are not satisfactory. It must be checked with Fit-Checker to avoid impingement (compression).

B) Case 2. Phonetic problem.

Despite the fact that the patient did not show the finish line on the gingiva, the patient claimed to have phonetic problems because "air escaped" through the interpapillary area.

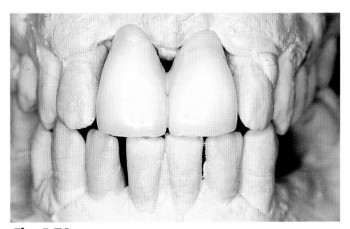

Fig. 5.74

The prosthesis returns from the laboratory with a diastema at the central papilla to facilitate hygiene.

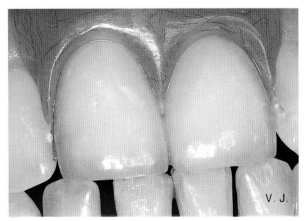

Fig. 5.75

Artificial gingiva placed in the mouth. Observe how it covers the mesial papilla of the neighboring laterals to improve phonetics.

5.5 Combination with natural dentition

A) Case 1. Lower prosthesis attachments.

In this case, we shall replace with implants the lower anterior teeth (right central and lateral, and left central, lateral, and canine), and the left second premolar and first molar. The natural canine is intermediate to the implants. The solution takes into account the loss of this tooth, so that the whole prosthesis will not have to be redone.

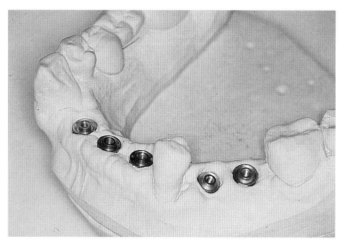

Fig. 5.76

Cast model of the case, with three standard abutments in the lower anterior and two in the left posterior area. These latter two had good alignment, so they were changed for tapered abutments to improve posterior esthetics.

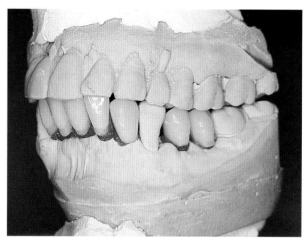

Fig. 5.77

Prefabricated teeth are mounted to check esthetics, and a silicone index is taken to facilitate anterior waxup afterward.

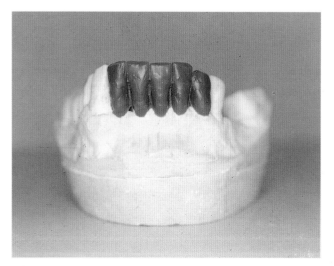

Fig. 5.78

Waxup is finished.

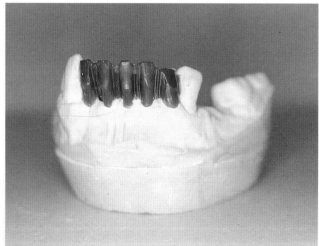

Fig. 5.79

Width is reduced evenly to achieve a good design of the framework for the porcelain.

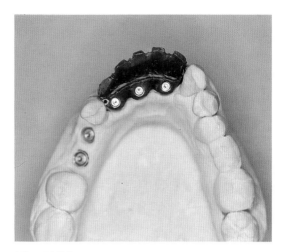

Fig. 5.80

The lingualized implants can be seen here, which is the reason we used standard abutments.

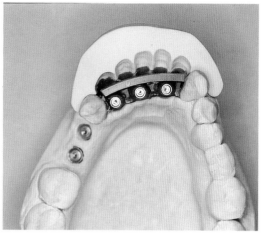

Fig. 5.81

The index is checked for sufficient space to place the porcelain without problems.

Figs. 5.82 and 5.83

Anterior metal framework try-in. At this time, we change the posterior standard abutments for tapered ones.

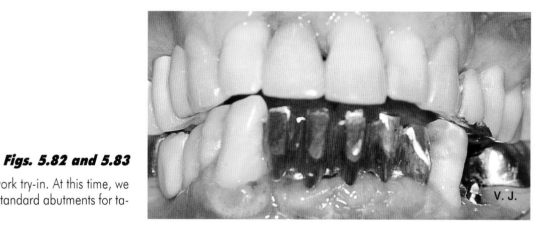

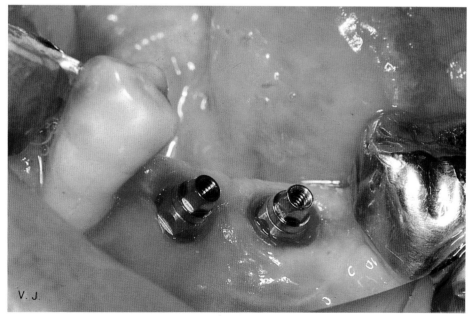

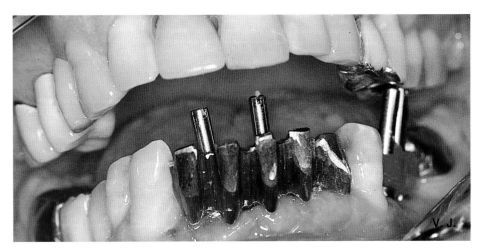

Fig. 5.84

Long screws are placed in the anterior for impression-taking. In the posterior area, transfer copings for tapered abutments (Estheticone) are placed and splinted.

Fig. 5.85

The impression is poured. The cast model shows the new posterior abutments.

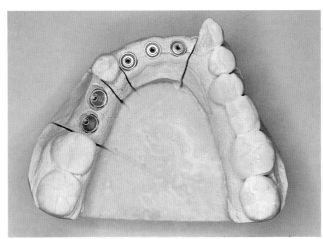

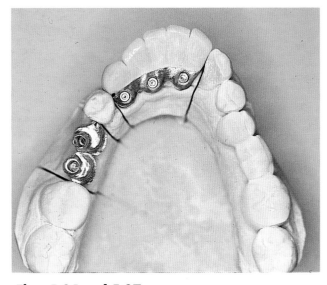

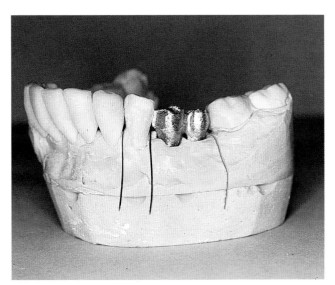

Figs. 5.86 and 5.87

Porcelain has been placed on the anterior segment; the metal structure can be seen on the posterior.

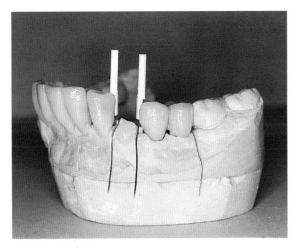

Fig. 5.88

Two female Plasta attachments (Cendre et Metaux) are placed in the design distal to the canine and mesial to the second premolar, eliminating the first premolar from the model.

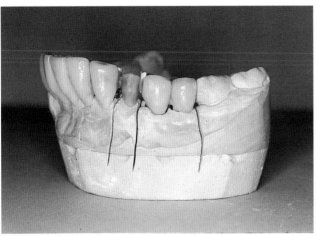

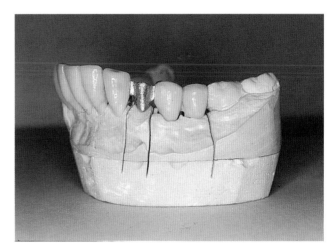

Figs. 5.89 and 5.90

Structural waxup of the corresponding first premolar, where the male of the two attachments is placed. We proceed to cast it.

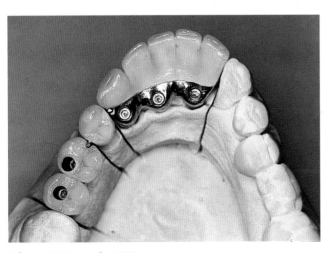

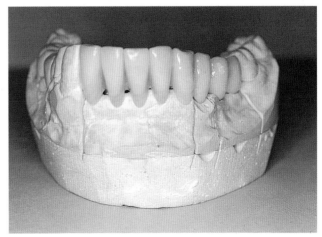

Figs. 5.91 and 5.92

Once the intermediate tooth is lost, this will be the definitive prosthesis. At least one of the attachments should be soldered.

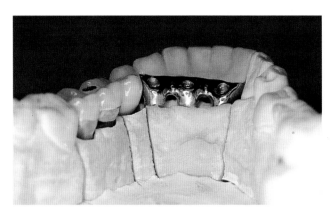

Fig. 5.93

Observe the lingual design for good hygiene.

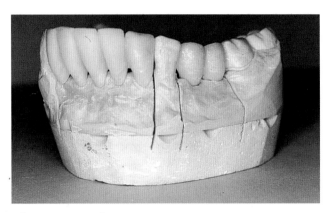

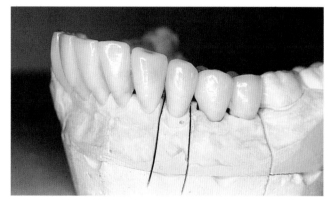

Figs. 5.94 and 5.95

Prosthesis with intermediate natural tooth and with the crown fitted into the attachments. Until the tooth is lost and replaced by the substitute, the female part of the attachments will be blocked out with composite resin to avoid food retention.

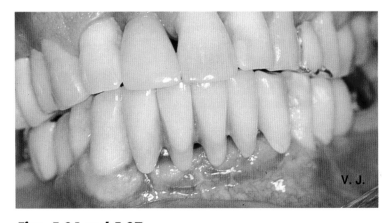

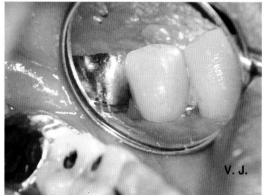

Figs. 5.96 and 5.97

Finished prosthesis placed in the mouth. Notice the wide embrasures between the second premolar and first molar.

In the following chapter we will describe posterior difficulties in depth.

V

B) Case 2. Upper prosthesis attachments.

Part of this case was presented in the section on angulated abutments in this chapter.

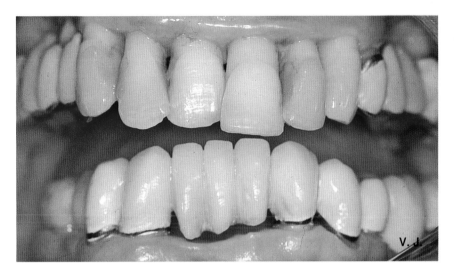

Fig. 5.98

The patient presented. After radiographic study, it was decided to save the upper right canine and second molar, as well as the upper left canine, and second and third molars. They were endodontically treated and reinforced with cast posts.

Fig. 5.99

Panoramic radiograph before implant placement.

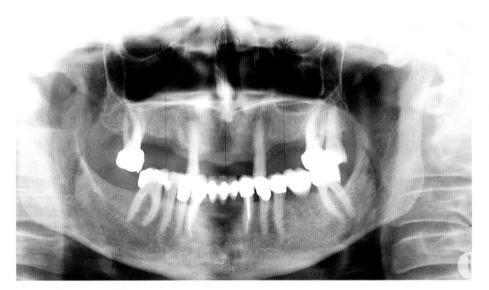

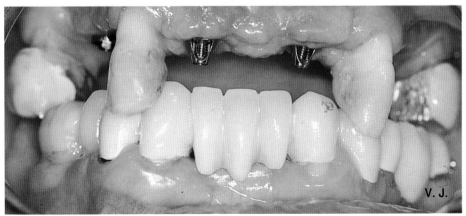

Fig. 5.100

Angulated abutments in the anterior area. Two standard abutments were also placed in both posterior areas.

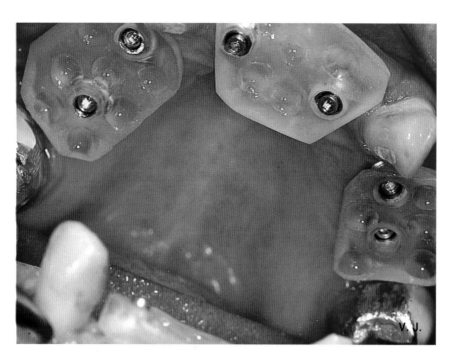

Fig. 5.101
Acrylic-resin stents placed for centric-relation registration.

Fig. 5.102
The prosthesis design was based on three sections over implants, crowns on the second molars, and crowns with attachments on the canines.

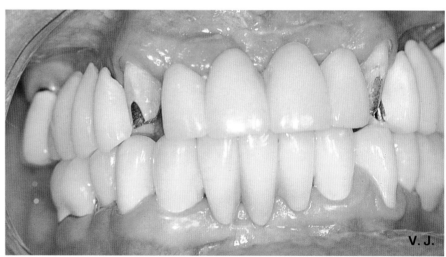

Fig. 5.103
Lingual view. The attachment distal to the canine can be seen. Should these teeth fail in the future, they could be easily soldered once the gingiva has readapted.

5.6 The Estheticone tapered abutment

A) **Case 1.** Fixed upper anterior restoration.

The Estheticone abutment will be further detailed in chapter VI, section 1.

We present a case of full restoration, focusing on the anterior area (to study the entire case, see chapter X).

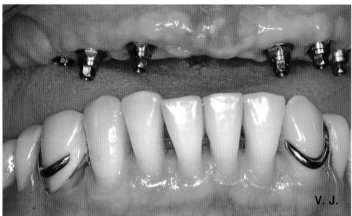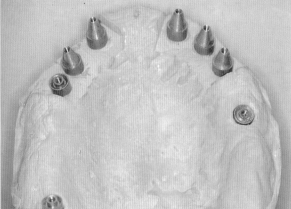

Figs. 5.104 and 5.105

The sites of choice to place the tapered abutments are the lateral incisors, when possible, to achieve good anterior esthetics. Special care must be taken to have an even anterior ridge to obtain good adaptation of the central incisors. The size of the Estheticone will depend on the needed 1- to 2-mm subgingival placement of the shoulder. This way, the tooth will emerge from within the gingiva, creating a natural-looking prosthesis.

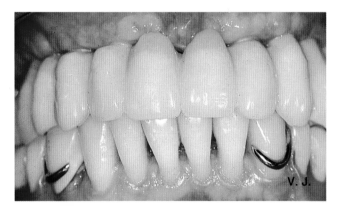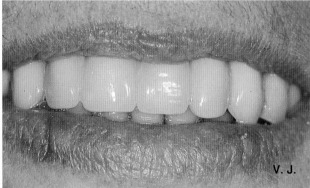

Figs. 5.106 and 5.107

Acrylic-resin provisionals are constructed to verify shape, color, and smile line.

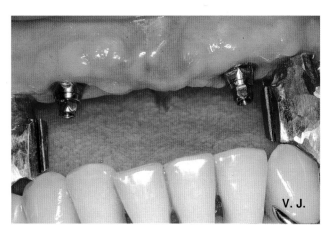
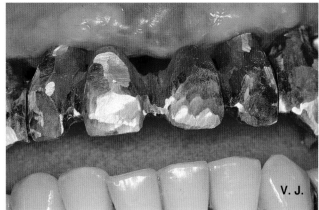

Figs. 5.108 and 5.109

The framework is cast in three sections. The anterior section (four incisors) will be splinted with attachments to the rest.

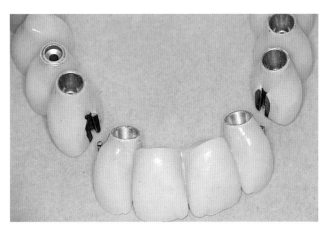
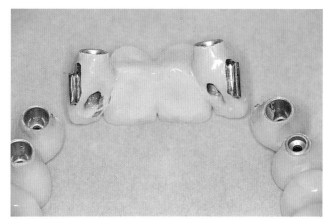

Figs. 5.110 and 5.111

Finished prosthesis, buccal and lingual views. Notice the five tapered abutments.

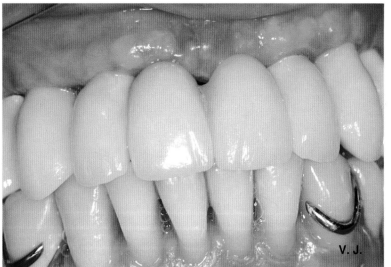

Figs. 5.112 and 5.113

Upper part finished and installed (see anterior section) and final panoramic radiograph.

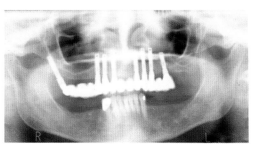

VI

POSTERIOR DIFFICULTIES:
PARTIAL PROSTHESES

Being able to construct partial prostheses, especially cantilevers, is one of the major advantages of implant treatment.

Nevertheless, it should not be forgotten that they have their indications and should not replace conventional fixed prostheses where warranted. This treatment modality is faster, less invasive to the patient, and has proven, through time, to achieve excellent results.

For example, if a first molar is missing, we would prefer to replace it with a conventional three-piece porcelain or gold prosthesis.

If all molars are absent, we have two options, depending on the nature of the opposing dentition and patient demands:

a) To prepare the two premolars and place a three-unit prosthesis, with the first molar cantilevered and shaped like a premolar.

b) To place two or three implants in the edentulous ridge and construct a two- or three-unit prosthesis.

If the second premolar is also missing, the only solution for using a fixed prosthesis would be an implant-supported one. The reason is that occlusion is needed at least up to the first upper molar to avoid TMJ tension. This situation would pose further difficulties if we had moderate periodontal problems with uncertain long-term prognosis.

The solution in these cases would be a prosthesis combining implants with telescopic structures, to be described later, or attachment solutions that would facilitate substitution of the missing posterior teeth. In other words, from a prosthodontic point of view, there are several situations:

— Adequate implant position for prosthetic treatment.

— Lingualized implants.

— Inadequate implant inclination.

— Natural dentition and implant combination.

In this last case, and according to our philosophy, single implants are contraindicated for molars.

6.1. Favorable implant position: tapered abutments

When an implant is in a favorable position, that is, well-placed in the ridge, tapered abutments (Estheticone) are recommended.

These abutments, as their name indicates, are conical, and at the base they present a subgingival shoulder.

This helps us achieve tooth emergence from within the gingiva, thus achieving good esthetics and facilitating patient oral hygiene.

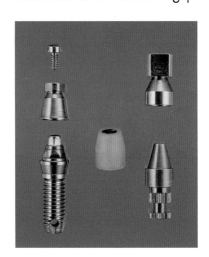

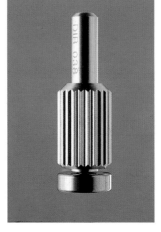

Fig. 6.1

The left picture shows the tapered abutment and how it relates to the implant. The healing cap is found in the center, with the impression coping and gold analog to the right. Above this, we have the gold cylinder that will be included in the prosthesis and the gold screw, normally hexagonal, that will join both structures.

Fig. 6.3

Manual screwdriver to check Estheticone fit on the implant.

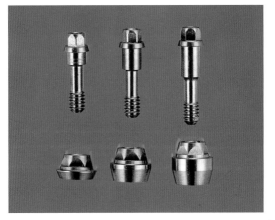

Fig. 6.2

The tapered abutments are available in several lengths (1, 2, and 3 mm); the selection will be determined by gingival height and subgingival shoulder placement. They are usually placed 1 to 2 mm subgingivally.

A) **Case 1.** Wide embrasures.

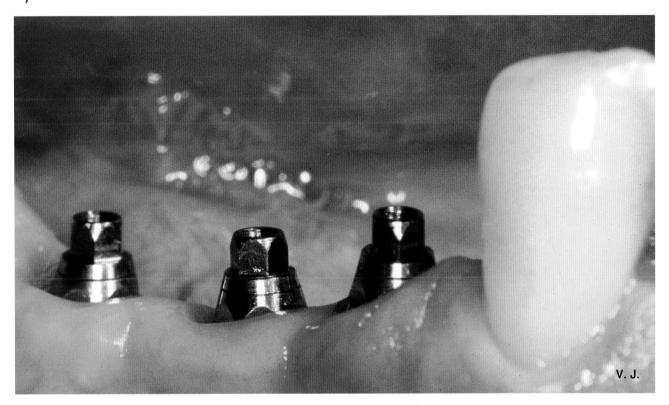

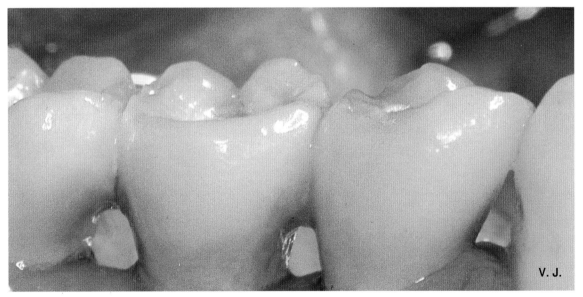

Figs. 6.4 and 6.5

Lateral view of tapered abutments installed in the mouth. Notice the wide embrasures, which were possible because there was sufficient space with respect to the opposing dentition.

B) Case 2. Insufficient space between arches.

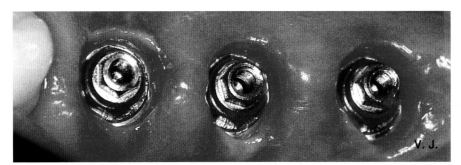

Fig. 6.6

Occlusal view of tapered abutments. Observe the subgingival shoulder.

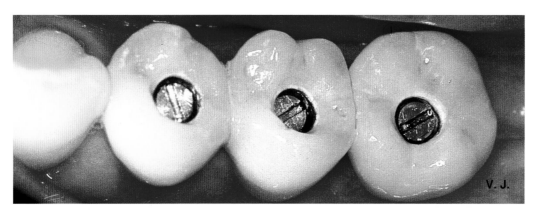

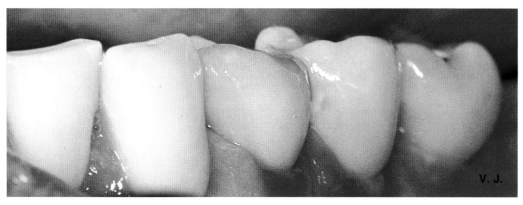

Figs. 6.7 and 6.8

Prosthesis placed in the mouth. The screws emerge at fossa level in the three units. This favors composite resin placement, thus achieving physiological occlusion.

Hexagonal screws may be used; however, in this case because of lack of space, flat ones were used.

The prosthetic teeth emerge from the gingiva as if they were natural teeth.

C) Case 3. System, clinical, and laboratory procedure description.

As seen previously, good esthetic results, function, and oral hygiene can be obtained; the following is a step-by-step description of how to construct a prosthesis over tapered abutments.

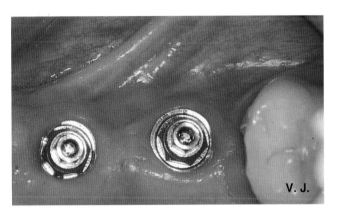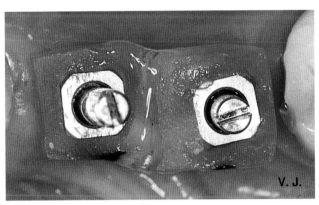

Figs. 6.9 and 6.10

Tapered abutments and specific impression transfer copings in the mouth. Posterior access is difficult, so shorter screws are used. These are splinted in the mouth with Duralay or light-cured acrylic resin.

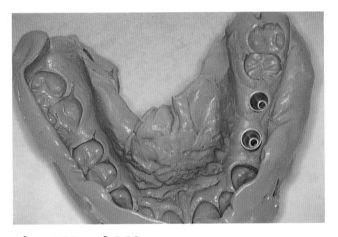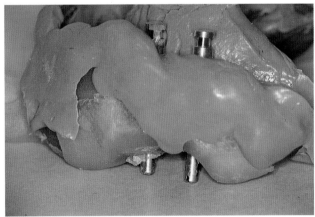

Figs. 6.11 and 6.12

The impression is taken with a customized tray from the laboratory that has an opening over the implant site. Soft wax is placed over it to allow unscrewing and removal.

The specific analogs are placed, as seen in the picture, and screwed to the transfer copings. The next step is to pour the impression.

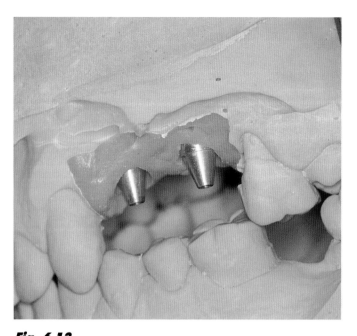

Fig. 6.13

Cast view of the tapered replicas and subgingival shoulder.

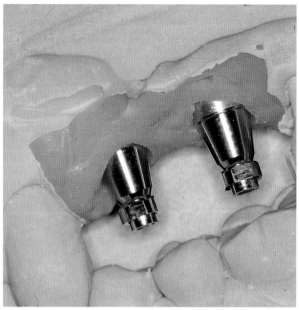

Fig. 6.14

Now we place the gold tapered abutment cylinders over the analogs in the model.

The case has been mounted previously on the articulator so we can verify the relationship with the other arch and the space available. Should there be insufficient space, opposing occlusal surface reduction would be needed.

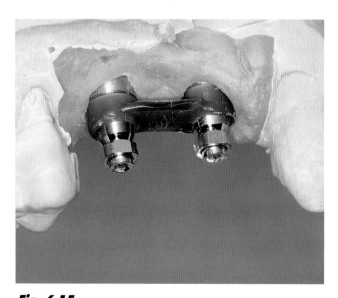

Fig. 6.15

The waxup is started (see chapter XII). A uniform platform, splinting the two cylinders, is covenient for wide embrasures.

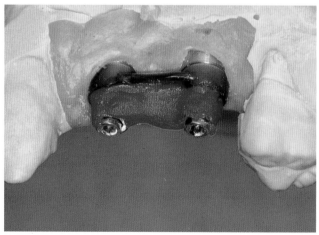

Fig. 6.16

To avoid wax distortion when removed, the gold cylinders should be splinted with Duralay. Afterward they are sectioned again to avoid contractions, and they are rejoined. They should remain like this for 24 hours.

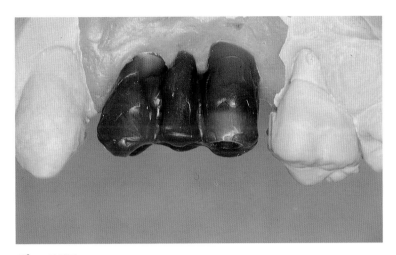

Fig. 6.17
The cylinders are joined with wax and modeled to the desired framework form and later cast.

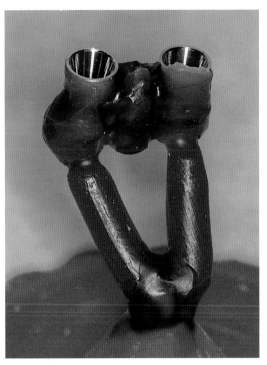

Fig. 6.18
Prepared sprues.

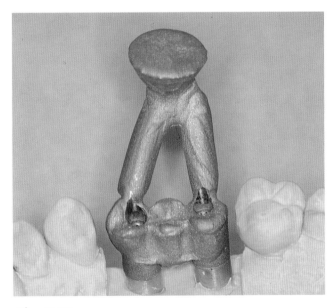

Fig. 6.19
Finished cast.

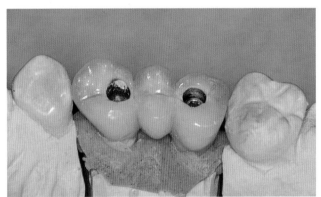

Fig. 6.20
Once the cast has been polished, the opaquer is placed, followed by dentin and enamel. The occlusion is checked.

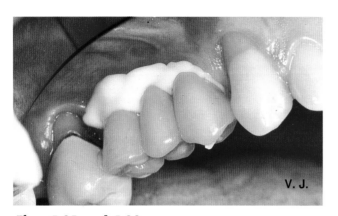
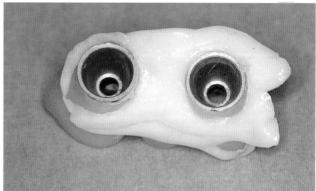

Figs. 6.21 and 6.22

It is placed in the mouth with Fit Checker to see if there is gingival impingement which would need relief.

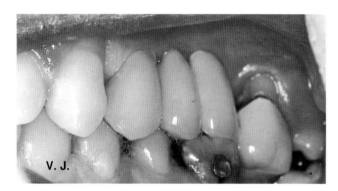
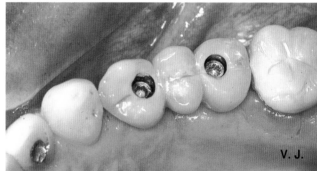

Figs. 6.23a and 6.23b

Prosthesis installed. Lateral and occlusal view.

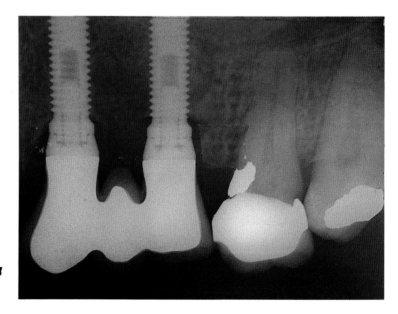

Fig. 6.24

Radiograph to verify fit.

D) **Case 4.** Natural dentition and implants without splinting.

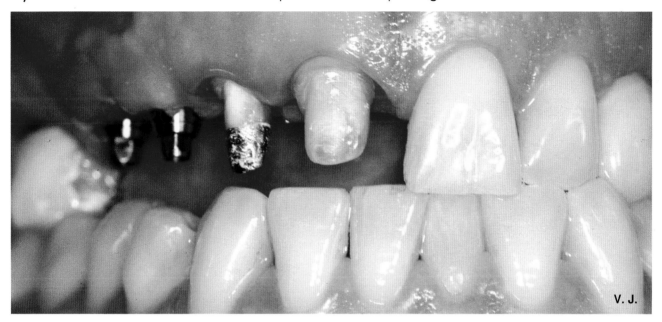

Fig. 6.25

Upper right central and lateral incisors are prepared for conventional porcelain-fused-to-metal crowns. At the canine and premolar area we have two tapered abutments.

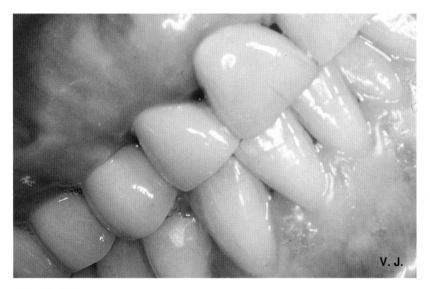

Fig. 6.26

Case completed, with an implant-supported prosthesis in the canine-premolar area. Disocclusion will be carried out by the incisors.

6.2 Unfavorable lingually or palatally positioned implants: standard abutments

A) Apparent contours technique

This situation refers to very lingualized or palatalized implants that make esthetics difficult to achieve.

In these cases, standard cylindrical abutments are used, combined with the technique we have named "apparent contours." This consists of creating an optical illusion to obtain good esthetics, yet allowing for good hygiene.

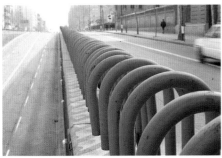

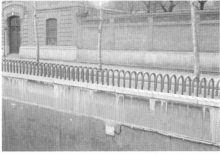

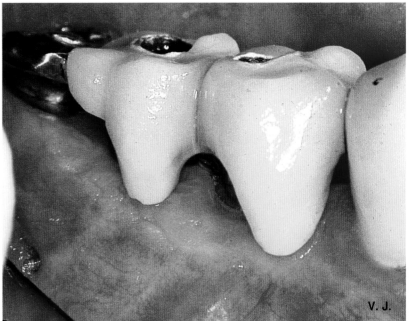

Figs. 6.27 and 6.28

Our goal is to have a continuous, solid surface when viewed anteroposteriorly, which will, however, on a lateral view have wide embrasures that can be fully penetrated with an interproximal toothbrush.

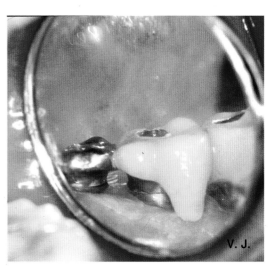

Figs. 6.29 and 6.30

When viewed anteroposteriorly, the implants cannot be seen, yet on a lateral view there is easy access to them.

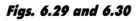

A.1. **Case 1.** Clinical and laboratory procedure description.

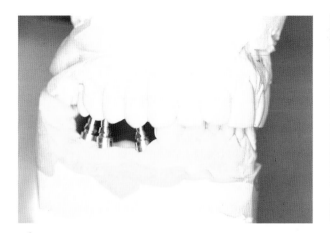

Fig. 6.31

The central implant will determine prosthesis contour; the other two implants are too lingualized.

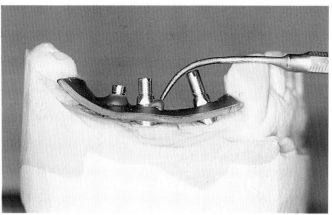

Fig. 6.32

Once the gold cylinders have been tightened, we proceed to construct a wax base evenly separated from the gingiva.

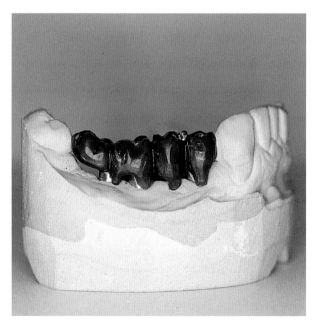

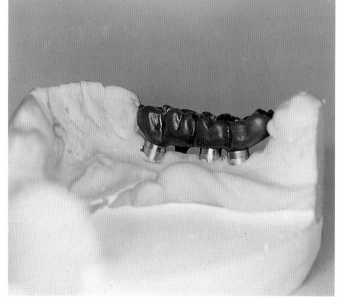

Figs. 6.33 and 6.34

The waxup is completed, creating drop-like mesial structures to hide the implant and to simulate natural root anatomy.

From the lingual, we can observe in better detail the open areas that flow evenly for good hygiene.

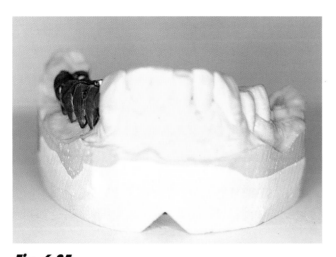

Fig. 6.35

The anteroposterior view shows that none of the implants is visible.

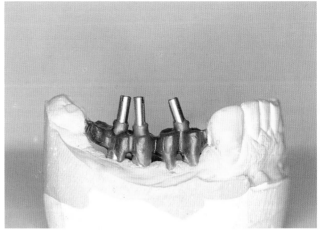

Fig. 6.36

The wax is cut back to gain enough space for porcelain placement, leaving the screw housing and drop-like mesial extensions.

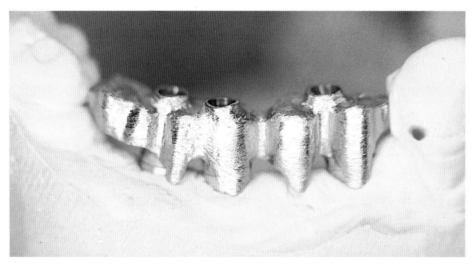

Figs. 6.37 and 6.38

Metal framework once cast, from the buccal and lingual views.

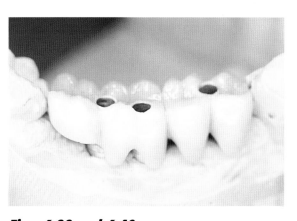
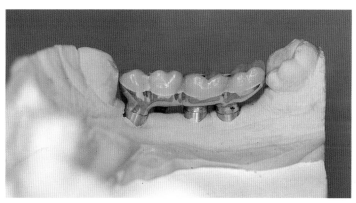

Figs. 6.39 and 6.40

Final completed prosthesis with porcelain, from the lateral and lingual views.

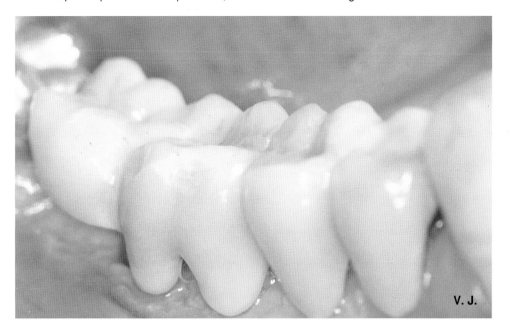

V. J.

Figs. 6.41 and 6.42

Prosthesis placed in the mouth and screw housing blocked out with composite resin.

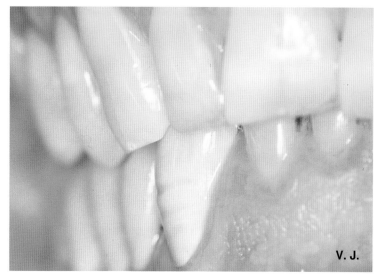

V. J.

6.3 Inadequate implant inclination: angulated abutments

Inclined implants will force the screw housing to be located on the buccal or on an active cusp; here the use of angulated abutments is indicated (see chapter V).

A) **Case 1.** Cantilever unilateral lower prosthesis.

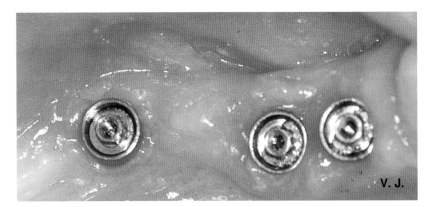

Fig. 6.43

Three implants placed in the mouth. The two anteriors are slightly lingualized, but the distal is far to the buccal.

Fig. 6.44

The provisional shows a posterior crossbite that the patient feels uncomfortable with from cheek biting. For this reason, we decided to exchange it for an angulated abutment.

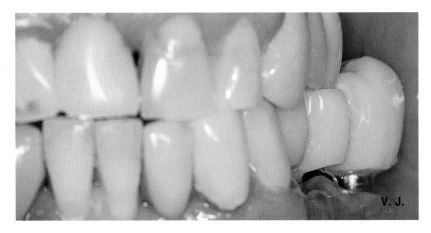

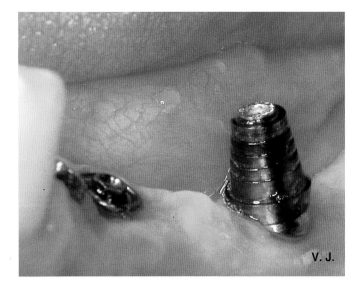

Fig. 6.45

The angulated abutment has been placed. The provisional system consists of plastic male and female sections, so as to modify the provisional and verify the new occlusion and anatomical form (see chapter XI).

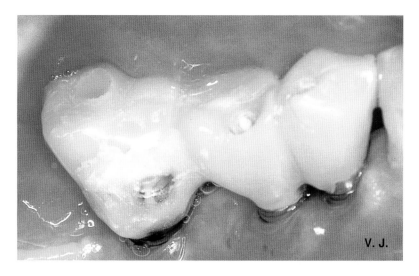

V. J.

Fig. 6.46

Notice that thanks to the angled abutment we have reshaped the provisional and reduced the occlusobuccal surface.

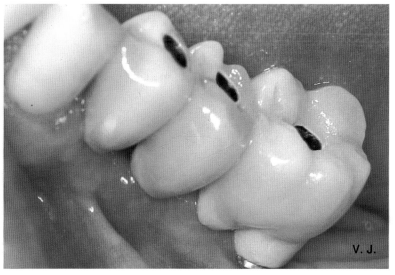

V. J.

Figs. 6.47 and 6.48

Case completed. Here we can observe that the screw exits were placed at fossa sites, and the occlusion with the opposing tooth has been physiologically improved.

V. J.

6.4 Combination of natural dentition and implants with intermediate teeth

Depending on implant position, standard or tapered abutments will be used, employing the corresponding prosthetic technique.

A) **Case 1.** Telescopic crown solution.

Let us analyze a case with a missing lower second molar and first premolar on the same side. The intermediate teeth (first molar and second premolar) were periodontally involved with furcation involvement and poor prognosis. In spite of being treated by a periodontist, personal hygiene was not too strict. The patient, however, wished to save these teeth at all cost. Two implants were placed in the edentulous segments.

Since we do not recommend single molar implants, our goal was to splint them and seek a future solution to the loss of intermediate teeth, without having to reconstruct the prosthesis.

It was decided to endodontically treat the teeth and use telescopic crowns in the interimplant segment.

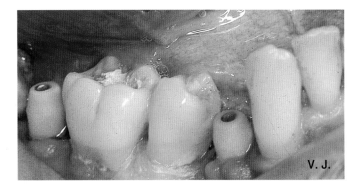

Fig. 6. 49

The two Estheticone abutments, with protective caps, are placed. The intermediate teeth have been endodontically treated; notice the plaque on the lower left first molar.

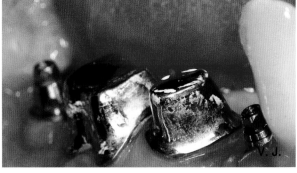

Fig. 6.50

Telescopic crowns are cemented with Panavia. The two tapered abutments can be seen without their protective caps.

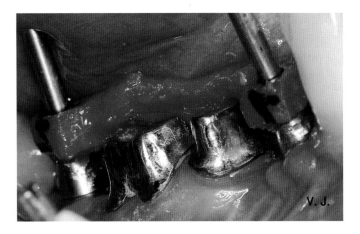

Fig. 6.51

Both impression copings are splinted above the telescopic crowns.

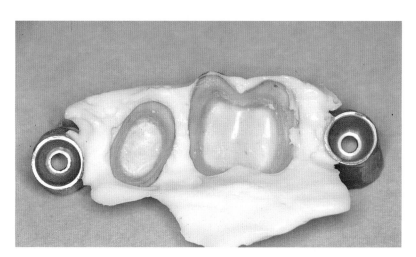

Fig. 6.52

Once the prothesis is completed in the laboratory, the fit is checked in the mouth with Fit Checker (quick-setting hard silicone).

Fig. 6.53

The prosthesis installed. Observe how the furca of the first molar is relieved and the screw exit emerges at the fossa area. The intermediate area was cemented with Nogenol.

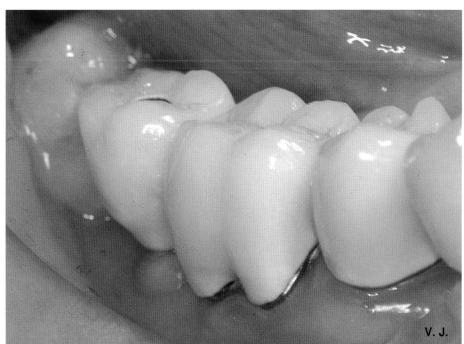

V. J.

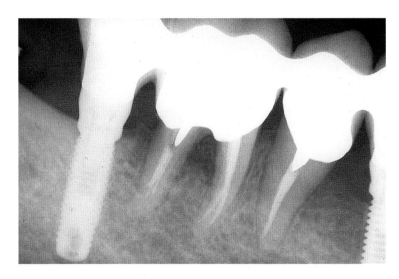

Fig. 6.54

Radiograph to check the prosthesis fit. The third molar has been extracted. Should the natural teeth fail (notice the furcation involvement), the same prosthesis can be readapted. In some cases, radiographs have shown intrusion of the intermediate teeth after several months. It is therefore advisable to incorporate screws laterally in order to fix the telescopic coping to the prosthesis structure.

6.5 Combined prosthesis over anterior natural dentition and posterior implants

A) Case 1. Prosthetic solution with attachments.

Full restoration: overdenture over four upper implants, in combination with natural teeth, in the lower anterior area and bilateral posterior edentulism; three implants were placed on both sides.

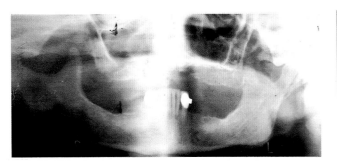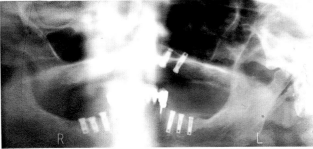

Figs. 6.55 and 6.56

Panoramic radiographs before and after implant placement. It was decided to retain the lower left canine and the lower right canine and first premolar. They were endodontically treated and reinforced with cast dowels.

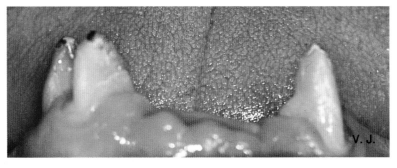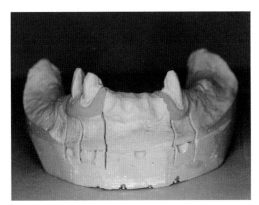

Figs. 6.57 and 6.58

Mouth preparation and master model in the laboratory with soft tissue model around abutment teeth.

It has not yet been established how to combine natural teeth and implants, with or without splinting. In this case, the implants will support the anterior teeth, because it is useful to have natural teeth serve as anterior guidance. This philosophy will be exercised in cases with adequate periodontium, because proprioception is extremely important in lateral excursions.

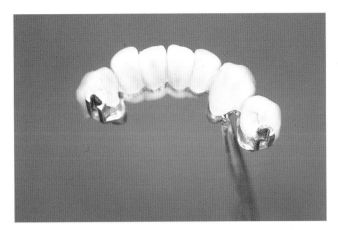

Fig. 6.59

Prosthesis design. A ledge has been prepared distally and a CM Box (Cendres et Metaux) matrix placed.

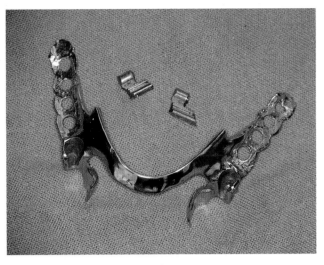

Fig. 6.60

Lower removable metal framework that the patient will wear until implants in both arches osseointegrate.

Notice the sheath to which the distal portion of the attachment will be cemented.

Fig. 6.61

Lingual view of the installed prosthesis.

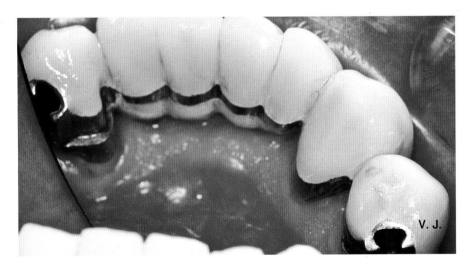

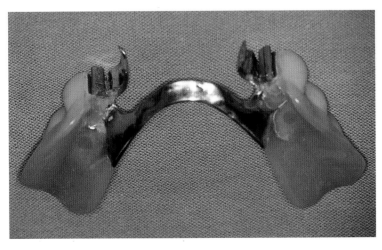

Fig. 6.62

Removable prosthesis completed with the patrix attachment positioned and cemented in place.

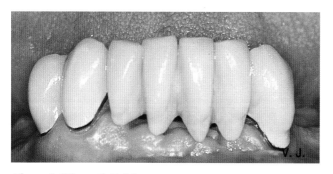

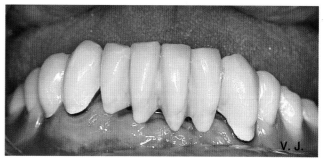

Figs. 6.63 and 6.64

On left, buccal view of fixed prosthesis. On right, removable and fixed prostheses installed.

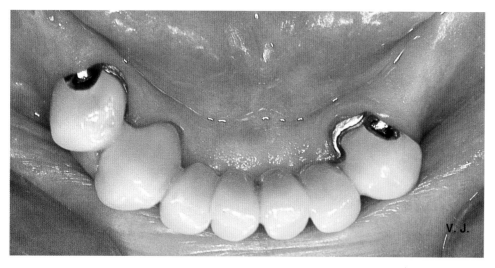

Figs. 6.65 and 6.66

View of the lower-arch fixed prosthesis with and without implants. Six standard abutments were placed.

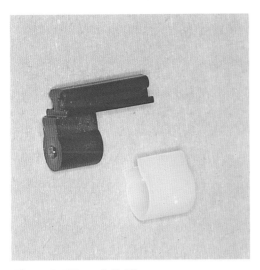
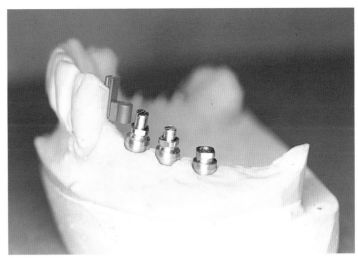

Figs. 6.67 and 6.68

Implant impression technique requires that the matrix of the attachment have a red patrix analog placed, so that once the impression is poured the attachment-implant relationship is in its precise place, thus allowing master model precision. This is later waxed up, including the analog, and cast.

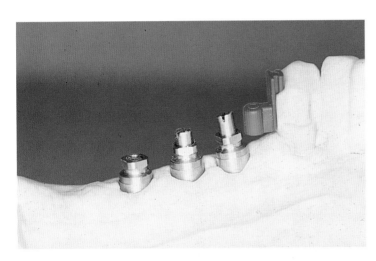

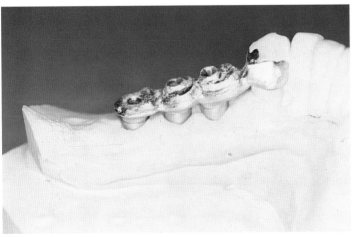

Figs. 6.69 and 6.70

Lingual view of the complex before and after casting. Notice the milled ledge created on the canine.

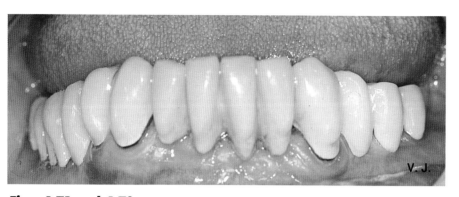
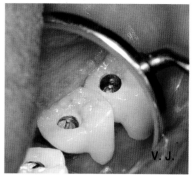

Figs. 6.71 and 6.72

Mouth view of prosthesis over implants. On the lower right side, the "apparent contours technique" was used.

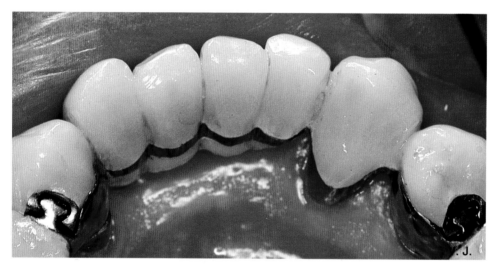

Figs. 6.73 and 6.74

Lingual view where the milled ledge for attachments can be seen joined to natural teeth. This will prevent their future extrusion.

The perfect design will also serve for good hygiene.

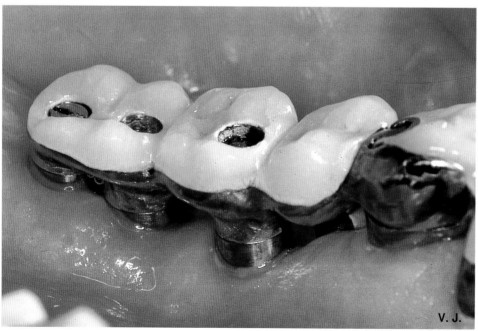

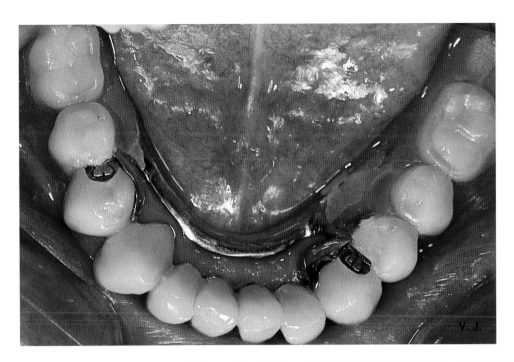

Figs. 6.75 and 6.76

Lower case before and 9 months after placing implant-supported prostheses.

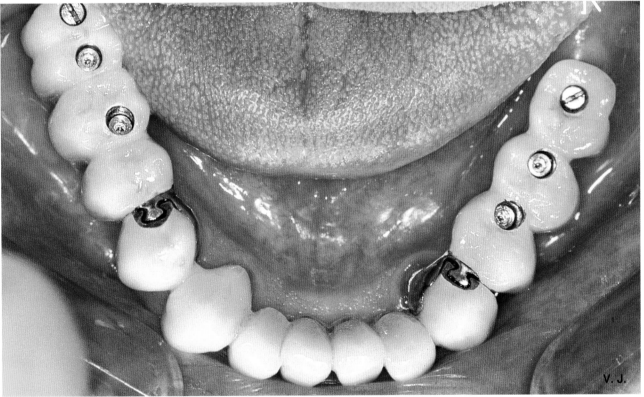

In some instances, natural teeth can be intruded, so the attachments selected must have some leeway, to permit without difficulty their return to their initial position. A screw attachment may be used to fix natural teeth to the implant-supported prosthesis.

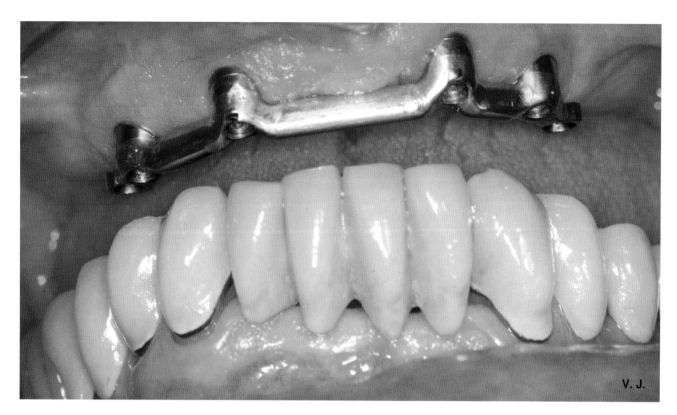

V. J.

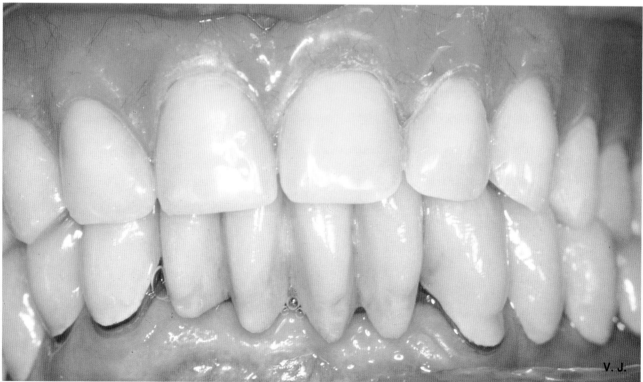

V. J.

Figs. 6.77 and 6.78

Case completed. The upper bar-and-attachment-supported overdenture, over four implants, was finalized 2 months after the lower.

6.6 Combining the three types of abutments

A) Case 1. Angulated, tapered, and standard abutments.

Finally, we are going to describe a case in which different abutments were used over three implants: one angulated abutment in the mesial, a tapered abutment in the intermediate, and a standard abutment in the distal. Should an implant be placed in the pterygoid process, a standard abutment is preferred, because it is more easily handled in this posterior location.

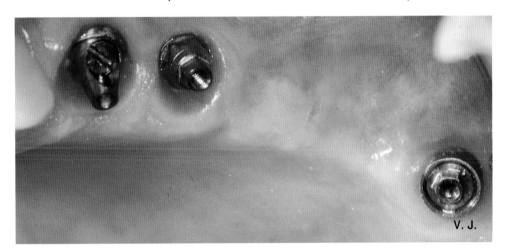

Fig. 6.79

View of the three different types of abutments in the same case.

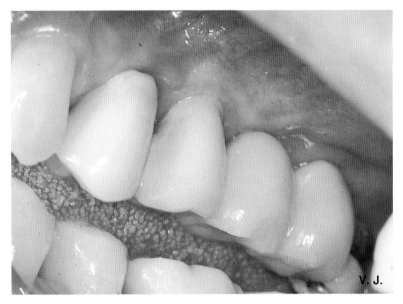

Fig. 6.80

Final prosthesis. Notice that the third molar hardly has any anatomy. In the first premolar a minute dark line can be seen gingivally due to an angulated abutment, which usually presents this difficulty. The second premolar emerges perfectly, because the shoulder is located subgingivally.

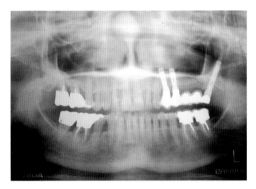

Fig. 6.81

Panoramic radiograph to control the fit. The length of the implants is adequate for a good prognosis.

In the near future, and despite good personal periodontal hygiene, new implant-supported prosthesis solutions will have to be devised in other dental segments.

6.7 Single posterior implants: CeraOne abutments

When referring to single posterior implants, only the premolars are considered, because, as previously mentioned, use of single implants in molars is not advised.

The only molar case accepted for single-unit implant-supported therapy is when two implants can be used, one in the mesial root and the other in the distal. These are splinted later through a single molar-shaped prosthesis.

A) Case 1. Single upper premolar.

We will describe the replacement of the first upper premolar using a CeraOne abutment and a porcelain crown over a flat alumina coping.

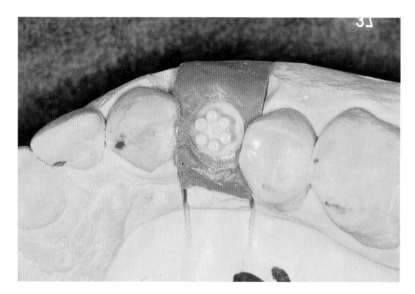

Fig. 6.82

Cast model, once the impression has been taken with the usual system and poured with its corresponding analog.

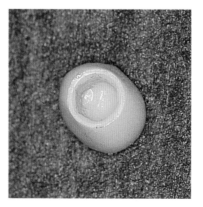 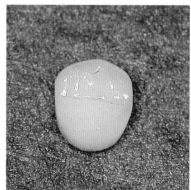

Figs. 6.83 and 6.84

Upper and lower views of the single crown. Notice the porcelain-free alumina shoulder and the reduced occlusal anatomy of the crown.

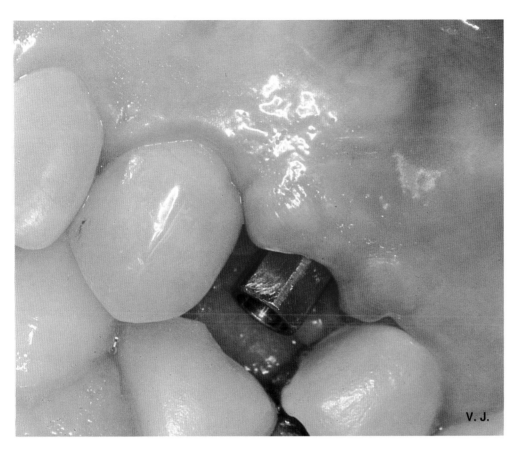

V. J.

Figs. 6.85 and 6.86

Before and after installation of CeraOne abutment and crown.

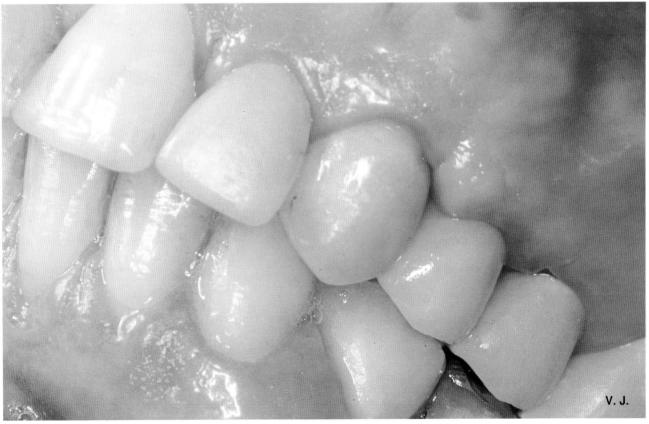

V. J.

VII

RESTORATIONS WITH NONCOMPROMISED VERTICAL DIMENSION

7.1 Introduction

Implant restoration in patients with compromised or noncompromised vertical dimension can be resolved through the following (see chapter I):

— Lower and upper overdentures.

— Lower and upper fixed prostheses.

While osseointegration is taking place, the provisional prosthesis plays an important role. It must be constructed in centric relation coinciding with maximum intercuspation, with perfect peripheral seal, good esthetics, and adequate vertical dimension. It should be relieved and relined with a soft material like Visco-gel.

On many occasions, the implants have osseointegrated but the patient's provisional restoration does not comply with these requisites.

In this chapter we will focus on the first situation, that is, a good provisional denture.

7.2 Denture duplication

The best information available to construct the final prosthesis is found in the patient's own prosthesis.

It provides:

— Vertical dimension.
— Centric relation.
— Tooth esthetics.
— Smile line.
— Peripheral ridge.

At the same time, it can be used as a customized tray, and initially as a surgical stent. The first thing to be done is to duplicate it according to the following technique (courtesy of Mr. Juan Carlos Delgado).

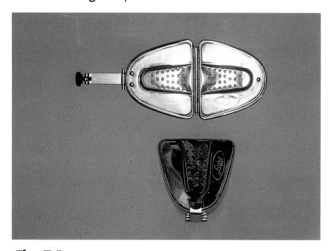

Fig. 7.1

Denture-duplicating device.

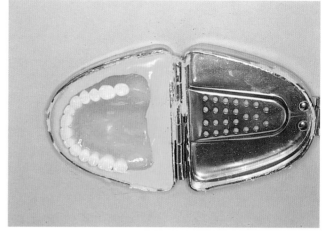

Fig. 7.2

Alginate is placed in one of the halves and the denture is pushed up to the edge. Once it has set, we do the same procedure on the other half, closing the duplicating device (the set alginate does not adhere to the fresh alginate).

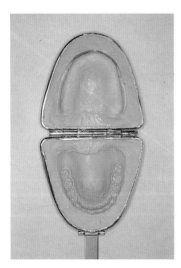

Fig. 7.3

Once the alginate has set, the device is opened and the denture is removed. The corresponding internal and external prints are then visible.

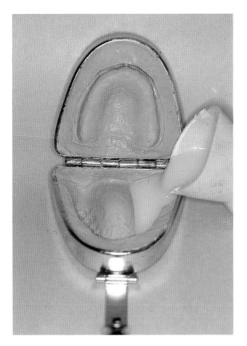

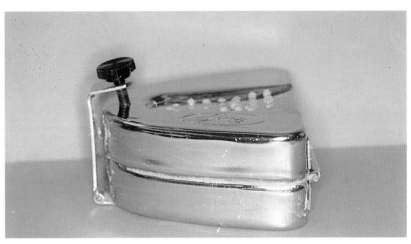

Fig. 7.5

The duplicating device is again closed and is put into a pressure pot with hot water at 1.5 atmospheres for resin polymerization. It is kept there 10 minutes.

Fig. 7.4

Self-curing resin is poured, filling the hollow surface.

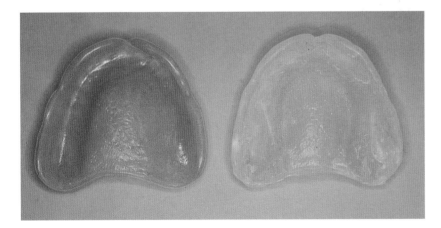

Figs. 7.6 and 7.7

Afterward, the polymerized resin is removed, the excess material is eliminated, and the copy is polished. This final result creates an exact duplicate of the provisional prosthesis.

7.3 Technical applications with case description

A) Case 1. Lower overdenture.

A lower implant-supported overdenture will be created. Before surgery, the prosthesis was duplicated and used as a guide for implant positioning.

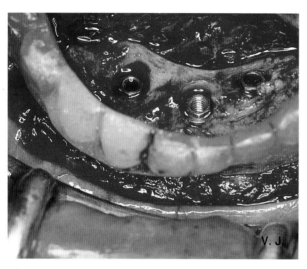

Fig. 7.8

Duplicate prosthesis used as a surgical stent during surgery (courtesy of Dr. Ramón Martínez).

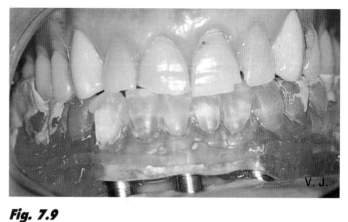

Fig. 7.9

Once osseointegration is confirmed, the prosthesis is duplicated again and used to check centric relation, which coincided (Blu-Mousse silicone was used).

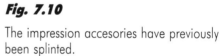

Fig. 7.10

The impression accesories have previously been splinted.

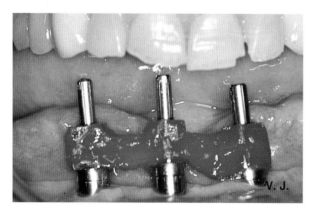

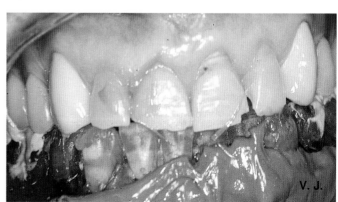

Fig. 7.11

The impression is taken, having the patient bite very softly to avoid disturbing the resilient capacity of the gingiva.

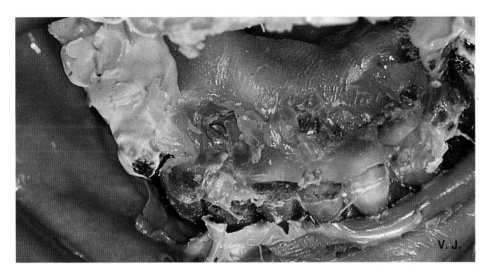

Fig. 7.12

An opening has been created in the duplicate, which is covered with soft wax so that the impression transfer copings can be loosened.

This is sent to the laboratory, and since all the information is available, the technician will be able to return the prosthesis almost completed. Perhaps we will only have to check bar adjustment, attachment anchoring, waxup for occlusal try-in, and peripheral seal. Almost all can be done in one appointment!

Fig. 7.13

Completed case.

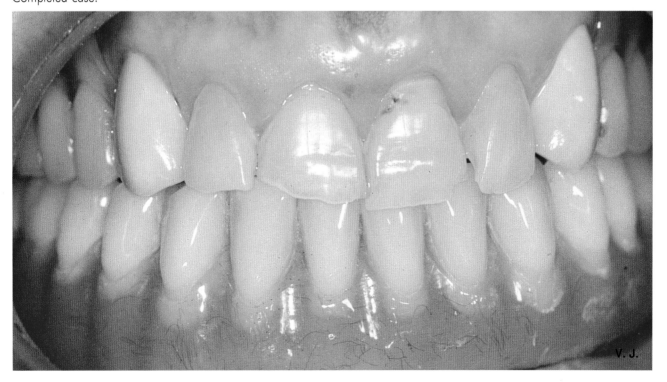

B) Case 2. Fixed lower prosthesis.

This patient was treated with an upper fixed prosthesis over natural dentition and a lower implant-supported fixed prosthesis.

The laboratory first constructed the upper fixed prosthesis, using as the opponent an impression of the removable prosthesis without implants. The patient's duplicate served as a customized tray.

The vertical dimension was left untouched because it was considered to be the correct one.

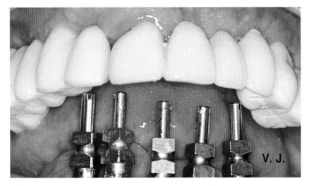

Fig. 7.14

Porcelain try-in in the upper arch. Impression transfer copings were placed on the lower arch and screws were selected.

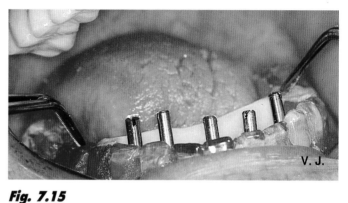

Fig. 7.15

Once splinted with Duralay, the duplicate is checked. Green resin had to be added to the lingual to widen the tray.

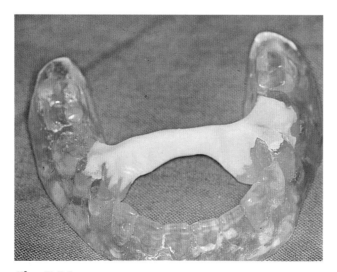

Fig. 7.16

View of the modified tray, due to implant lingualization.

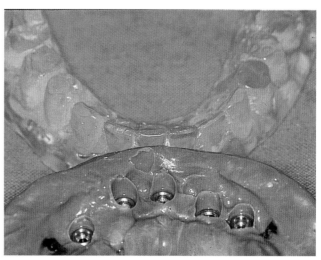

Fig. 7.17

Two duplicates were used in this case, one for the impression (modified) and the other as an occlusal reference.

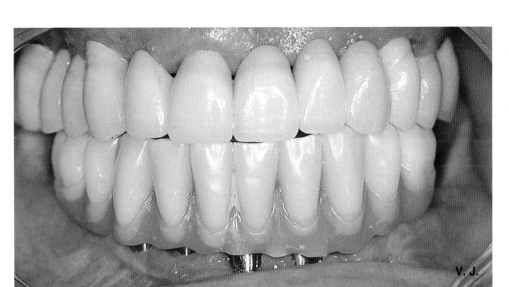

Fig. 7.18

Case completed and installed in one appointment. In the upper left there is a cantilevered premolar-shaped unit.

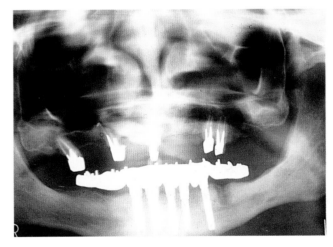

Fig. 7.19

Panoramic radiograph of the same case. Observe the length of the fixed lower implants which permitted the placement of two cantilevered units in the mandibular prosthesis.

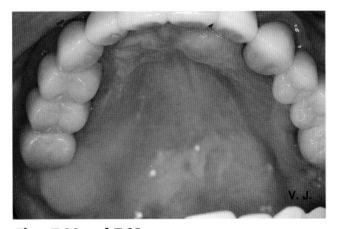

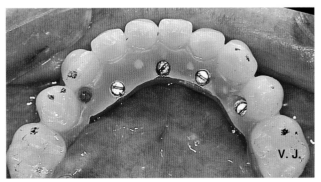

Figs. 7.20 and 7.21

Upper and lower occlusal views.

C) **Case 3.** Upper overdenture.

In this case, the patient wants equal denture esthetics.

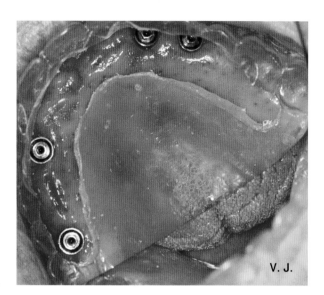

Fig. 7.22

The denture duplicate has been adapted to serve as an impression tray. Surface removal will be necessary in the upper left segment.

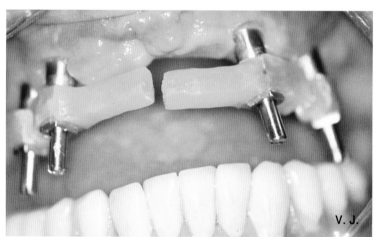

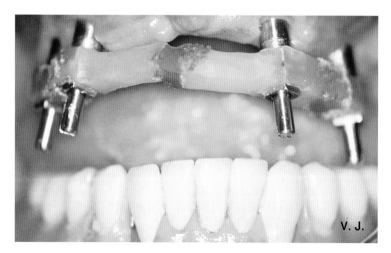

Figs. 7.23 and 7.24

The transfer copings come prepared from the laboratory, covered with acrylic resin and individualized. Afterward, they are splinted in the mouth with the same type of material or with composite resin (it seems to have less contraction).

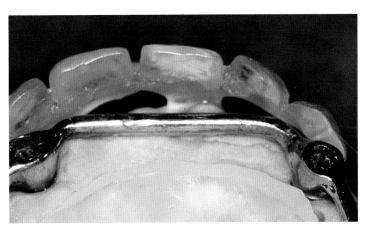

Fig. 7.25

The impression taken with the duplicate, serving as a customized tray, has permitted us to have some reference, once the bar has been constructed, as to how much buccal inclination will be needed for the canines. This will avoid a fragile surface that may fracture when in function.

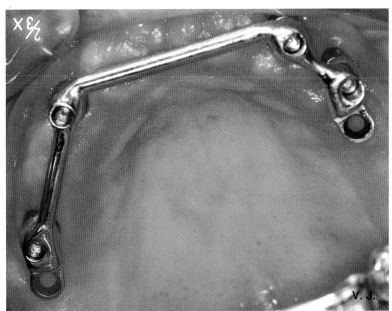

Fig. 7.26

The bar placed into position. Notice that resilient Ceka attachments were placed distally to avoid posterior prosthesis-loosening movement. The attachments will be active, for example, when the patient bites into a sandwich, thus producing forced leverage on the anterior teeth.

They have no function during mastication or in lateral movements because this is a mucosa-supported prosthesis and the attachments have resilience in all directions.

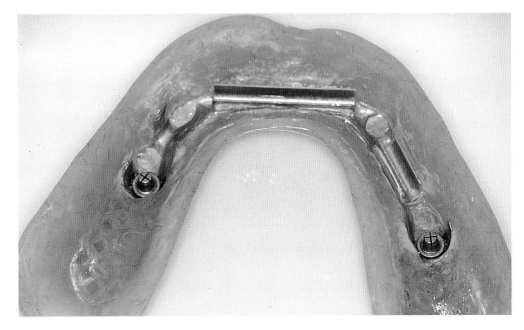

Fig. 7.27

Inferior view of the overdenture. The clip for the bar in the anterior and the posterior Ceka attachment can be activated. It should be emphasized that little palatal extension exists.

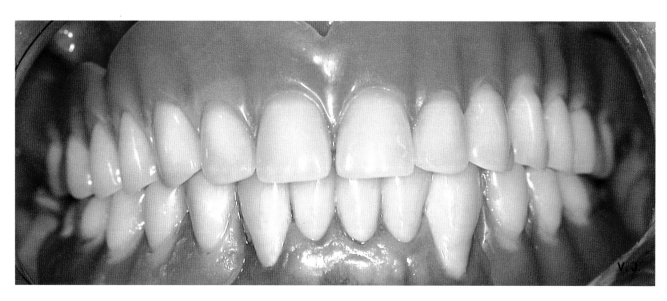

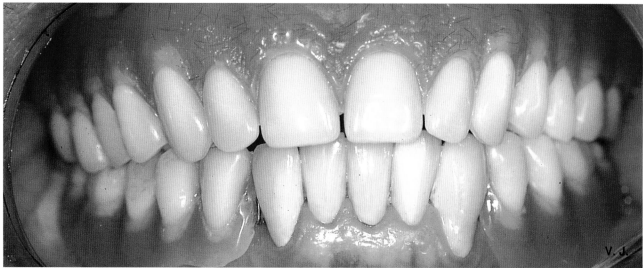

Fig. 7.28 and 7.29

Prosthesis before and after. The "forced" canine inclination can be seen. The rest is practically the same.

VIII

RESTORATIONS FOR COMPROMISED VERTICAL DIMENSION

8.1 Introduction

Compromised vertical dimension is the most frequently encountered situation. It is a result of tooth loss and old, ill-fitting dentures. This has also led to loss of centric relation and unpleasing facial esthetics, especially the lips and the nasogenial sulcus.

In these cases, we start from scratch and our effort should be guided to correct the profile; esthetics; and tooth form, size, color, and position.

8.2 Obtain intermaxillary registrations

A) In cases of bilateral posterior edentulism with implants

This is a very difficult situation due to contacts in the anterior only; when the patient bites hard this can pivot the mandible backward, giving us a false vertical dimension.

Althrough we can use maximum intercuspation as a reference for habitual occlusion, we must be sure it coincides with centric relation.

In cases of full restorations, we have designed some occlusal bite stents that serve two purposes:

1. They aid in verifying that the gold cylinders are correctly aligned with the abutments. Tension should not exist when they are installed and screwed in. This indicates that the impression was correct.

2. Since we have created a smooth surface with small grooves, we will be able to reposition the wax registration while mounting the case on the articulator. Its construction is very easy.

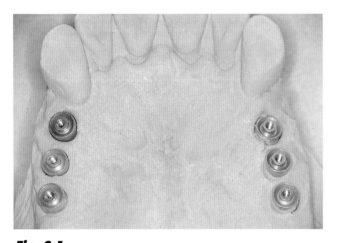

Fig. 8.1

Master model with three standard abutments on each side.

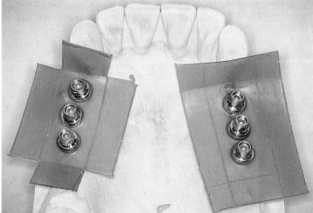

Fig. 8.2

The gold cylinders are screwed down and a small wax plate is placed, with the four corners cut out geometrically.

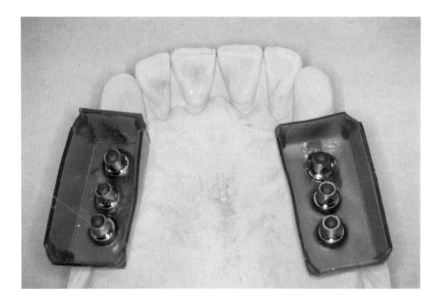

Fig. 8.3

The flaps are folded toward the center to make it look similar to a wax box.

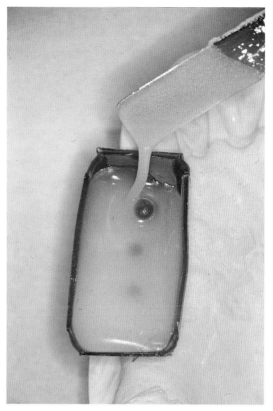

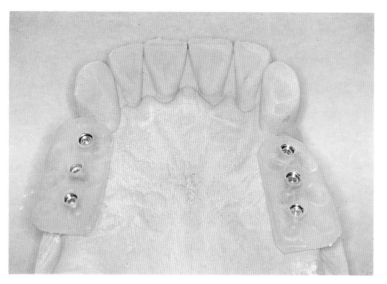

Fig. 8.4

Self-curing acrylic resin is poured into the box, with the access to the screws previously protected. It is allowed to set.

Fig. 8.5

Once it has been trimmed, we make rounded grooves on the occlusal face of the plastic stent and we proceed to clean out the access to the screws.

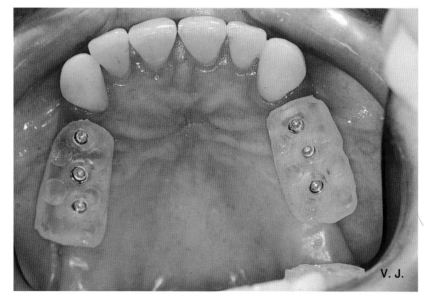

Fig. 8.6

It is placed in the mouth and the passive fit of the gold cylinders to the abutments is checked. The impression can be now considered correct. The design must take into account the width of the stent to avoid patient cheek-biting. It should also have the edges well-polished and the entry orifice to the screw wide enough to ease its placement.

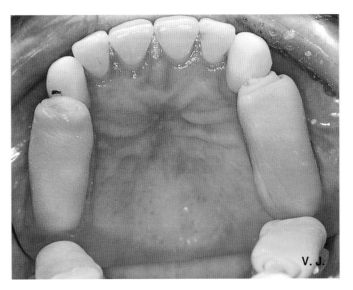
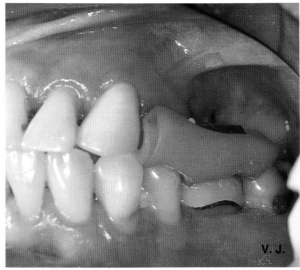

Figs. 8.7 and 8.8

A small roll of wax at 48 °C (Moyco) is set on the resin base and the patient closes gently while we guide the mandible to centric relation.

The wax is chilled with cold water and then removed from the mouth.

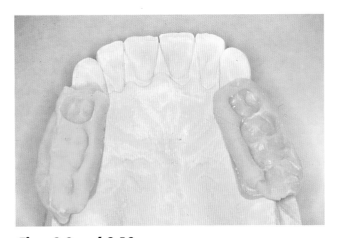
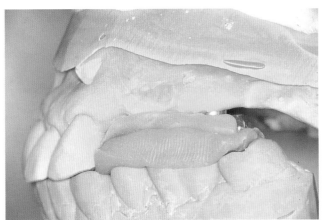

Figs. 8.9 and 8.10

The "bite plate" is screwed to the cast and the wax is placed over the grooves in the plastic.

The opposite arch is positioned and mounted on the articulator.

B) In total edentulism with implants

In these cases, it is important to determine not only the vertical dimension but also the smile line and the lip position that is most esthetic. These considerations must be visually checked with the patient in profile, frontally, and in centric relation.

We will not describe how to register the vertical dimension (the following is one method of doing it: muscular fatigue is induced by having the patient open wide, and once the mandible is back in the rest position, decrease 2 or 3 mm, corresponding to the neutral zone until we reach maximum intercuspation). In any event, each clinician can use the method that best suits him or her.

As explained in the previous section, "bite plates" are constructed but with a "plastic visor" to trace the smile line.

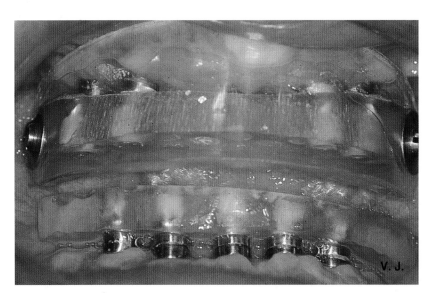

Fig. 8.11

In the top picture the "visor" held by lateral "clips" can be seen. This can be moved up or down and fixed in the desired position with a screw. The lower part will determine tooth length; in other words, the incisal edge.

The visors are constructed in different widths and lengths, and are interchangeable, which will permit us to select the most adequate for good placement or lip support.

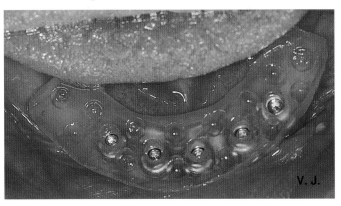
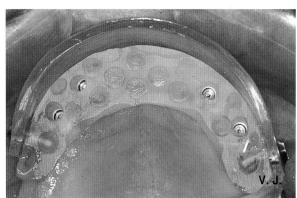

Figs. 8.12 and 8.13

On the left, wax imprints are shown. On the right, the visor and occlusal grooves are visible.

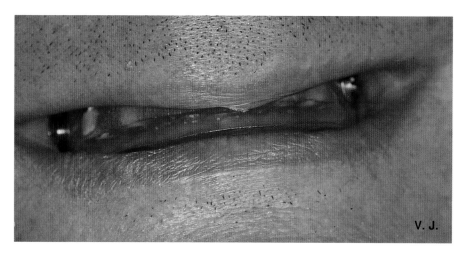

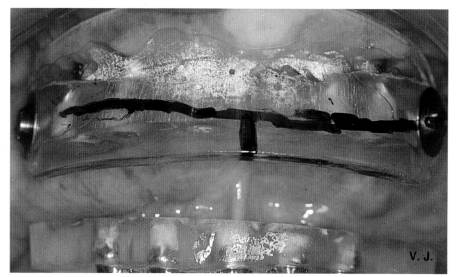

Figs. 8.14 and 8.15

Patient smile line, traced with a felt pen, and the midline.

Fig. 8.16

Centric-relation registration with appropiate vertical dimension.

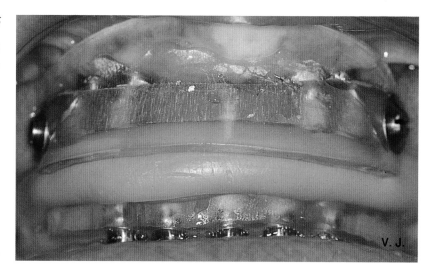

Since the "bite plates" are sturdy and are implant-supported, the occlusal references obtained are very reliable (mucosa resilience does not intervene).

C) In fixed upper implant-supported restorations with natural opposing dentition

In these cases the same technique is used, adding to it the acrylic-resin base, gold cylinders, and prefabricated teeth (chapter X).

8.3 Clinical case

Upper overdenture and lower fixed prosthesis, both implant-supported; clinical and laboratory procedure description.

In fixed lowers, hybrid prostheses are indicated. They consist of a one-piece metal rigid base, over which we place the acrylic teeth.

It is typical to have a patient come to the office, carrying pictures several decades old, who wishes to have the mouth restored as it was. It is a difficult task, but it is not impossible to achieve.

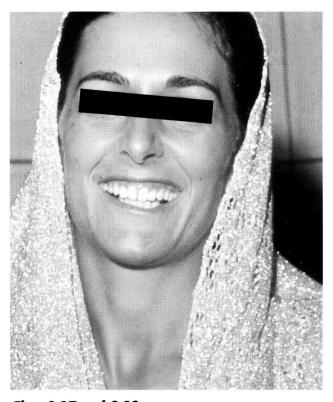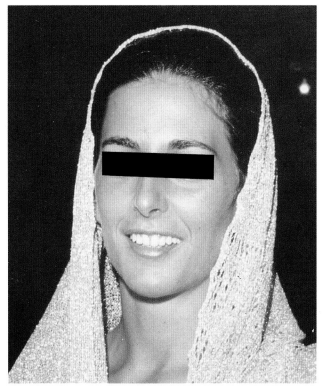

Figs. 8.17 and 8.18

These are pictures brought by a patient wishing to have her teeth restored to this condition. She was 20 years old when the pictures were taken.

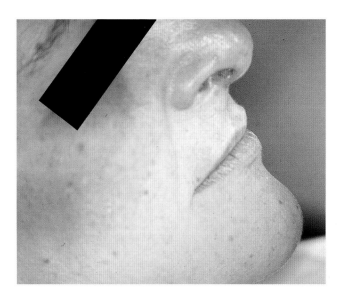

Fig. 8.19

The actual profile of the face showed a pronounced nasolabial angle, which made the nose look like it had dropped, and a nasogenial sulcus much accentuated, that made this good-looking patient appear older than her actual age. All of this was indicative of decreased vertical dimension.

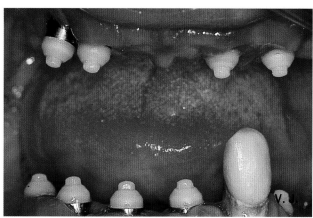

Fig. 8.20

The presenting case consisted of four upper implants (an overdenture was chosen for esthetics and because of lack of bone) and five lower implants, plus a retained canine of tremendous value for lower provisional-prosthesis support while osseointegration occurs.

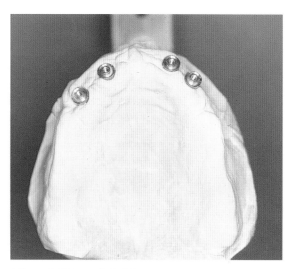
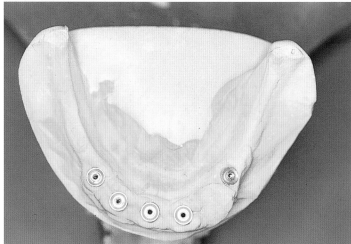

Figs. 8.21 and 8.22

The usual impressions are taken and poured, thus obtaining the master models.

Observe that the lower left canine has been eliminated.

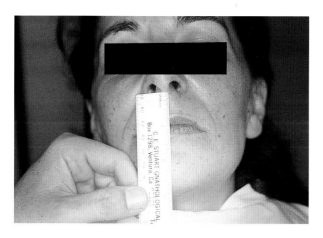

Fig. 8.23

Vertical dimension is registered, marking a dot on the chin in resting position, which will serve as a reference.

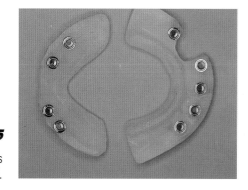

Figs. 8.24 and 8.25

The occlusal bite stents installed.

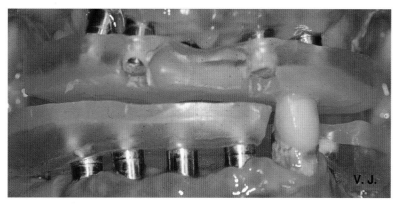

This stage is extremely important. We must make sure that the impressions are correct and that the fit of the cylinders is completely passive, because the day the prosthesis is installed, the canine will be extracted and there will be no turning back.

A variation has been introduced by placing wax on the occlusal face of the stent in the laboratory. This way, the cusp makes an imprint at the vertical dimension we are verifying with respect to the ruler measurements taken before.

The upper limit of the stent is adjusted to the smile line (by adding or removing acrylic resin) and checking the width to see if the lip is well-positioned, without needing to use a "visor" (see chapter VIII, section 2).

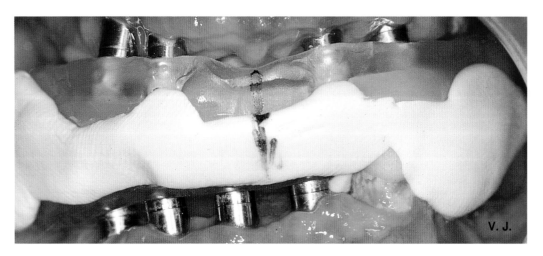

Fig. 8.26

The patient bites again into a hard-setting silicone just to the canine imprint registered previously.

The bite should not be forced so as to avoid TMJ pivoting.

The midline is also marked.

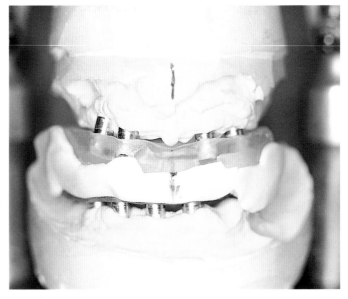

Fig. 8.27

Case mounted on the articulator.

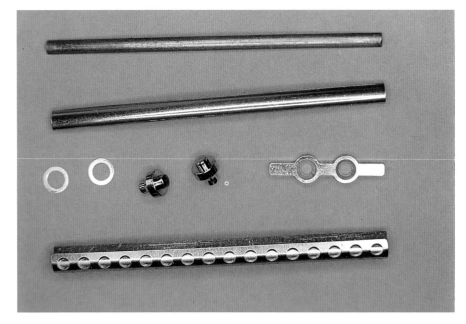

Fig. 8.28

Laboratory accessories for the upper (see chapter XII, section 3.6):

- Dolder bar.
- Ceka attachments.
- Resilient accesories.

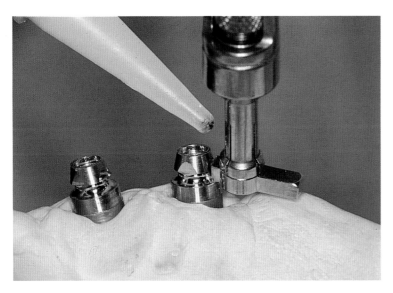

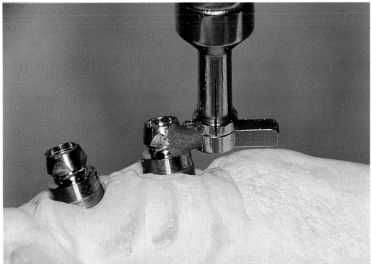

Figs. 8.29 and 8.30

The attachments are placed distal to the last implant with the surveyor.

They are glued with cyanoacrylate and fixed with Duralay. This is done on both sides.

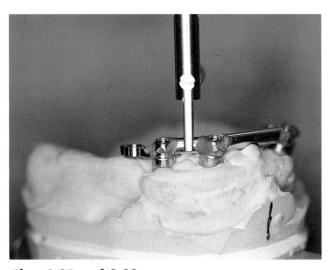

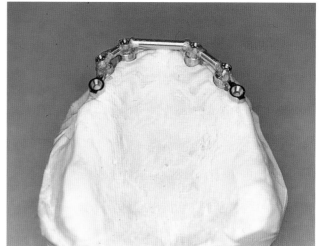

Figs. 8.31 and 8.32

The bars are placed the same way, linking the gold cylinders to each other.

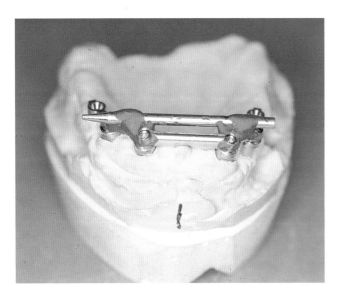

Fig. 8.33

Reinforcements are placed to avoid distortions while removing the complex from the cast model.

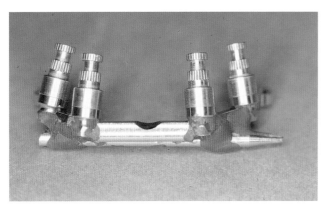

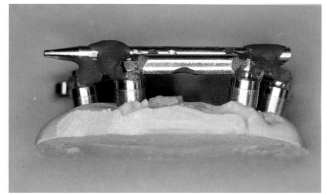

Figs. 8.34 and 8.35

It is removed from the cast model, the analogs are fitted, and it is poured, thus creating a new "working model."

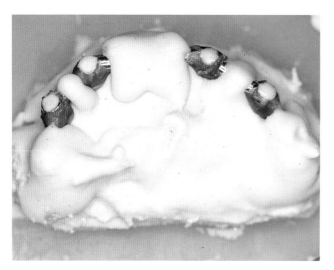

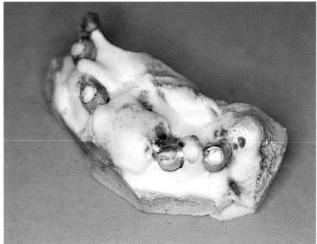

Figs. 8.36 and 8.37

The cylinders, bars, and attachments are invested and we proceed with the soldering.

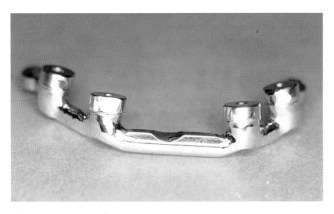

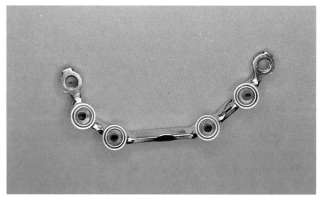

Figs. 8.38 and 8.39

The bar is completed (notice the cylinder protectors placed to avoid damage during polishing). The fit is checked on the model.

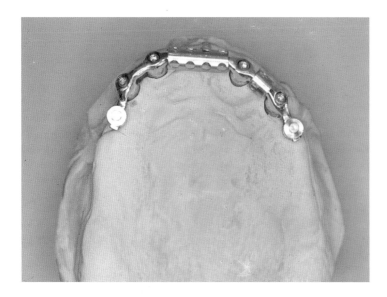

Fig. 8.40

Once the resilient elements are in place, the bar clips and the male parts of the attachments are seated. Sometimes, the corresponding anterior section is eliminated.

Fig. 8.41

Once the undercuts are blocked with wax, an impression is taken and poured. In this cast, we will proceed with the waxup of the future metal overdenture framework.

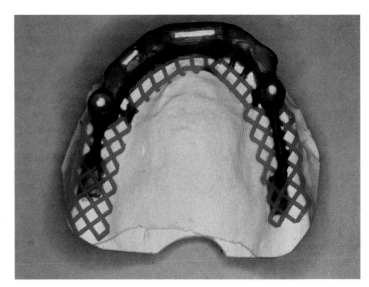

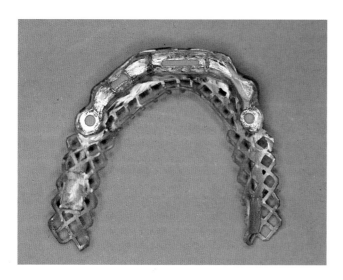

Fig. 8.42

Cast framework.

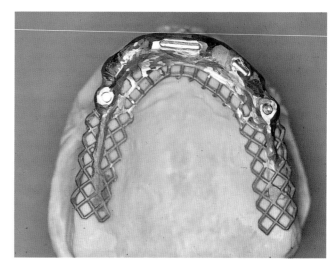

Fig. 8.43

The metal framework is placed over the clips and patrix of the attachments. The perfect fit can be seen here. Some internal elements exist to obtain resiliency.

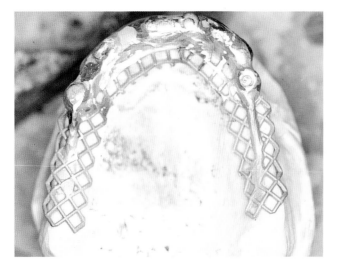

Fig. 8.44

Once the soldering is completed (structure, clips, and patrix), it will all be one piece.

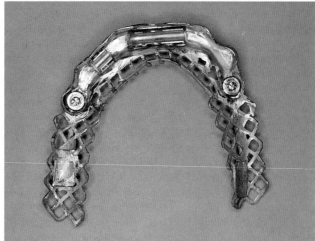

Fig. 8.45

Inner view of the complex.

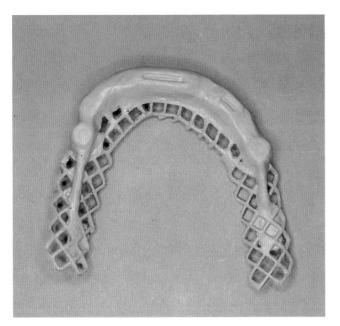

Fig. 8.46

Opaquer placement, followed by waxup and mounting of teeth.

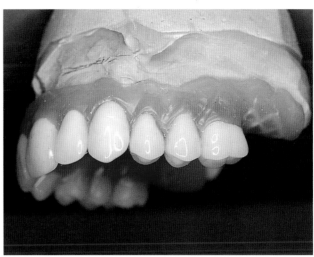

Fig. 8.47

Upper teeth mounted.

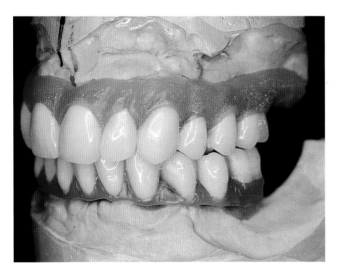

Fig. 8.48

Mounted upper teeth and lowers in the process of mounting.

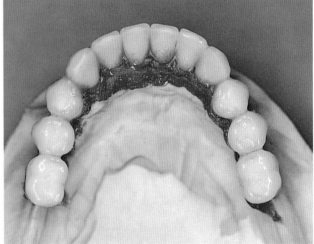

Fig. 8.49

Mounting of lower teeth is completed. It should be remembered that the first molar must be occluded.

Using this situation as a reference, the laboratory will design the lower metal framework (see chapter XII).

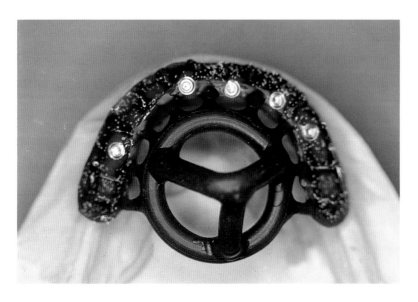

Fig. 8.50

Lower framework waxup ready for casting.

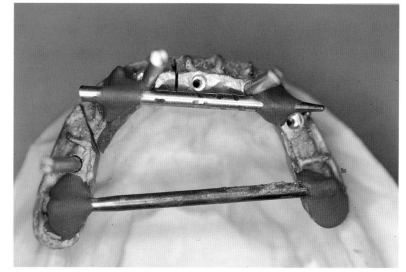

Fig. 8.51

When casting a curved structure, it is almost impossible to avoid distortion, which will make its fit problematic. In this case, the structure was sectioned and later soldered, following the technique described previously.

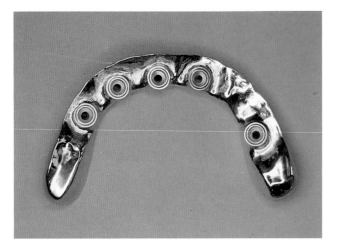

Fig. 8.52

Lower framework soldered and polished.

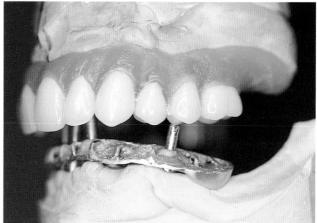

Fig. 8.53

Framework on the articulator.

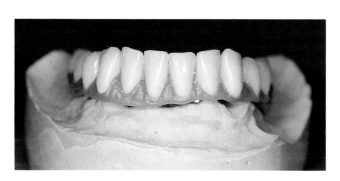

Fig. 8.54

Teeth are placed in wax on the framework following the occlusal imprints obtained beforehand during the first mounting of teeth (see chapter XII, section 3.3-B).

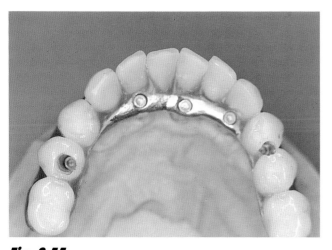

Fig. 8.55

Occlusal view of the lower framework with teeth mounted in wax. Notice the screw exit holes.

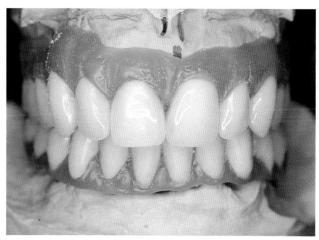

Fig. 8.56

Case mounted on the articulator with the occlusion adjusted.

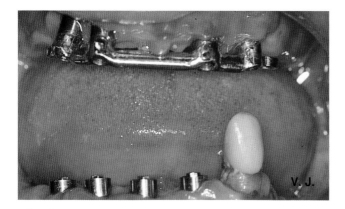

Fig. 8.57

The upper bar is installed to check fit. We then proceed to extract the canines.

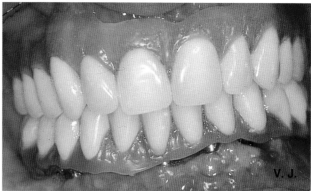

Fig. 8.58

The lower hybrid prosthesis is screwed to the abutments and the upper overdenture is positioned. We have the patient close in centric relation and verify that it coincides with maximum intercuspation.

Once it is acceptable, the prosthesis is sent to the laboratory.

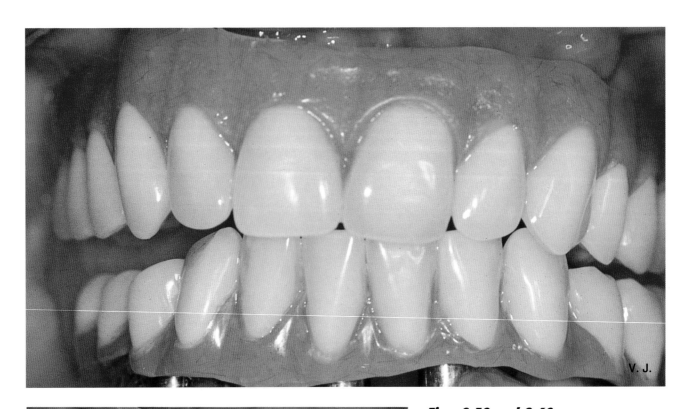

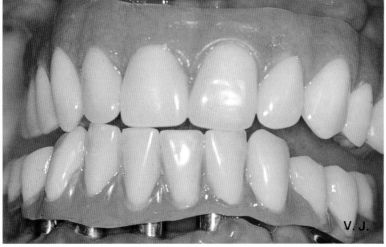

Figs. 8.59 and 8.60

When the restoration is completed, we check lateral and protrusive excursions.

As described in previous chapters dealing with occlusion, when the restoration consists of an upper overdenture and a fixed lower with sufficient implants, we prefer an organic occlusal scheme. During lateral excursions, the anterior teeth will be in charge of direction, eliminating any posterior contact. If retention is not adequate, we would have to consider a bilateral balanced occlusion.

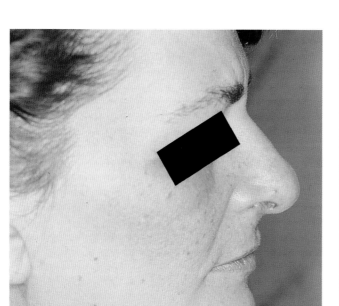

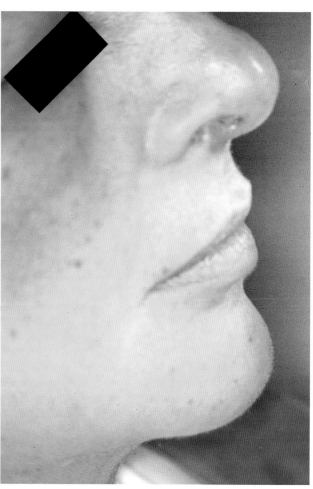

Figs. 8.61 and 8.62

Patient profile before and after. The nasogenial sulcus has diminished. The nasolabial angle has also improved and the nose is not so "droopy," since lip support has increased.

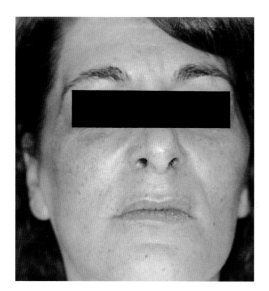

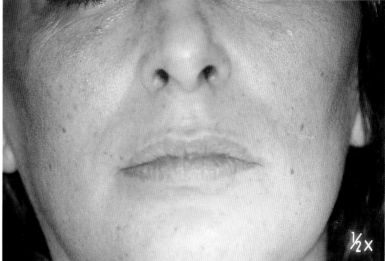

Figs. 8.63 and 8.64

Frontal view of the face where "excess lip" was present, and the pronounced nasogenial sulcus. Afterward, facial esthetics have improved.

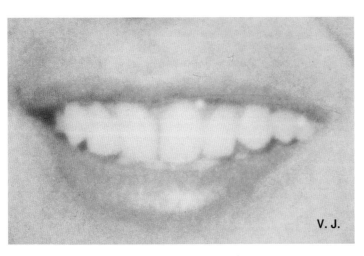

V. J.

Figs. 8.65 and 8.66

The smile from 20 years ago and the current smile are very similar with respect to gingiva and tooth form.

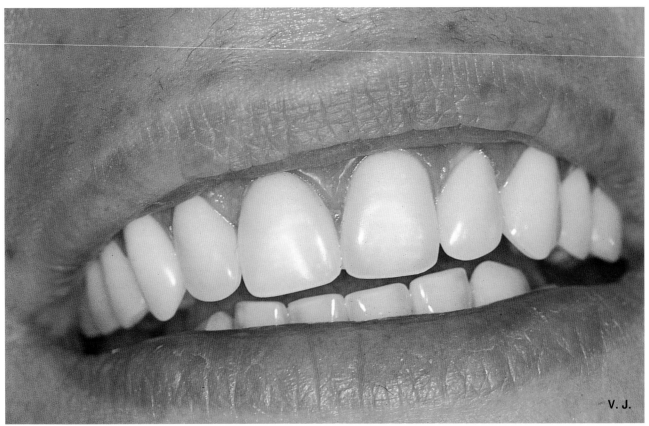

V. J.

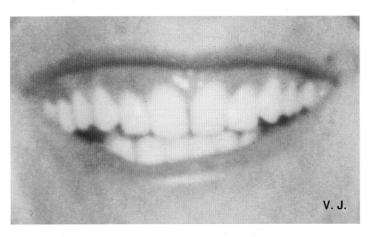

V. J.

Figs. 8.67 and 8.68

The broad smile shows the same gingiva and lower dentition.

Mission accomplished!

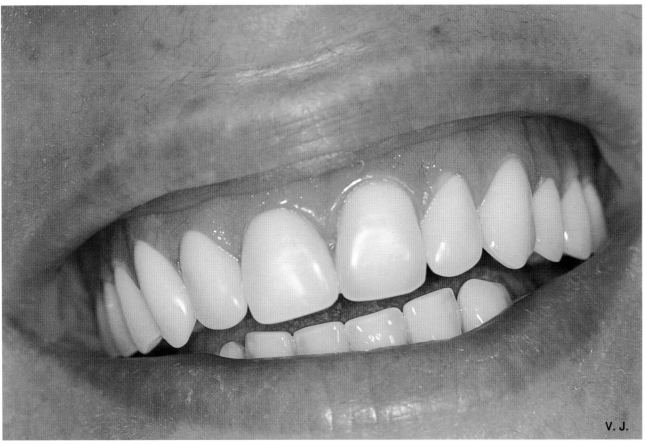

V. J.

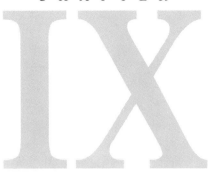

IMPLANT-SUPPORTED SCREW-RETAINED PROSTHESES AND THE CEMENTED COPING TECHNIQUE

9.1 Lower fixed restoration: hybrid prostheses

A) Technique description

With this technique, our goal is to have a perfect fit of the prosthesis over the implants, that is, to have the gold cylinders fit on the abutments to avoid negative tensions.

If we cannot have this, the forces will concentrate on one point (the only contact between the previously mentioned components, because of their flat surfaces), thus leading to increased bone loss.

The only way to avoid this, with respect to prosthesis construction, is through an absolutely passive fit.

Until today, and due to the difficulty in obtaining total precision in cast curved frameworks, it was almost impossible to have an initial perfect fit, which is why the framework was sectioned and soldered.

There were also various problems associated with the techniques of overcasting gold cylinders on wax structures.

Siirila et al (1988) proposed a technique by which the cylinders were joined by acrylic resin in the mouth and later the whole structure was overcasted.

Parel (1989) joined the first and last cylinder with a bar. The rest was integrated to the prosthesis through acrylic resin, but until the metal portion was complete, there was a fragile area.

To avoid these problems, we devised a framework design that is cast in one piece, without soldering, and that only incorporates the gold cylinder that will be used as a reference during installment.

The areas that will correspond to the remaining cylinders are prepared for later cementation in the mouth with anaerobic resins. These have previously been positioned and fixed to the transepithelial abutment. The exact relationship between the gold cylinder and the abutment is optimal, thus obtaining a perfect implant-prosthesis interrelationship.

The type of material that can be used in the mouth as a cement, with enough working time and the necessary adhesion to resist occlusal forces and saliva, is an anaerobic resin (Panavia).

Jörneus et al (1992) studied the maximum occlusal forces that appear over implants. The result was a variable average between 140 and 390 N. Adhesion strength studies using Nimetic (Espe), Panavia (Cavex), and Microfill Pontic (Kulzer) resulted in average values of 941 N at 10 minutes, reaching 1535.4 N and 1246.3 N at 24 hours. These values, after 4 months in contact with artificial saliva, were 2404.3 N, more than necessary to resist the forces that occur in the mouth.

Panavia was difficult to adhere to precious metals. This was solved by mechanical retention, oxidation, and contact surface tin-plating. A 3-year experience has shown that a passive-fit prosthesis is possible. This also simplifies laboratory procedures and achieves excellent results more reliably and faster than before.

B) Advantages, materials, and disadvantages

Advantages		Materials	Disadvantages
• Simple and quick technique. • In case casting fails, the framework and the gold cylinders are not lost. • Convenient polishing. • One-piece framework without soldering prevents bimetalism, which causes ionic changes. • Bimetalism is avoided through acrylic-resin isolation of the framework from the implants. • Lack of abutment tensions. • Uniform cylinder-abutment contact leads to balanced forces; in other words, a perfect fit. • Precision is repeatable in all cases. • Standard material available now can be used. • In case of cylinder debonding, it can be easily and accurately repositioned in the mouth.	• Should any of the implants fail, they can be repositioned in a larger-diameter cast model on the same bed, and after osseintegration occurs again, the cylinder can be repositioned by simply changing coping inclination, if necessary. This avoids reconstruction of the prosthesis.	• In these cases, Bråne-mark implants, Nobelpharma prosthodontic accessories, anaerobic acrylic resin (Panavia), noble silver-palladium alloy, and Duralay can be used. • Panavia was chosen as the adhesive material because: a) It is easy to handle in the mouth, since it is an anaerobic acrylic resin with sufficient working time. b) It maintains and increases adhesion in the presence of saliva. c) Sandblasting and tin plating improve its adhesion to noble metals.	• Porosity at the joint area. • Lack of long-term experience(3 years).

C) **Case 1.** Lower hybrid prosthesis cemented to screw-retained prosthesis over implants (for more details see chapter XII, section 12.3.3.b):

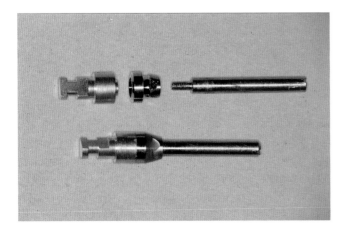

Fig. 9.1

The mechanical undercut is blocked out with wax at the level of the gold cylinder.

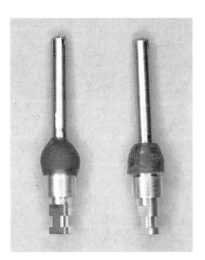

Fig. 9.2

Resin caps are constructed to adapt to the cylinders. These can be removed easily.

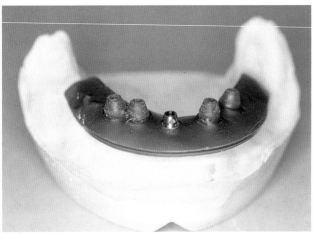

Fig. 9.3

The base of the framework is built up in wax, including the central gold cylinder and four caps without cylinders.

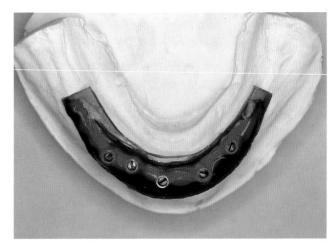

Fig. 9.4

The caps are splinted to each other with Duralay. Note that through the top of the caps we have access to the gold cylinders that are placed beneath, but they are completely free, except for the central that is included in the structure.

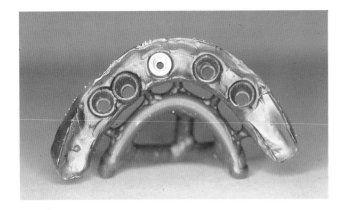

Fig. 9.5

View of the sprued and waxed-up framework, where we can clearly see the central cylinder and four lateral chimneys or caps.

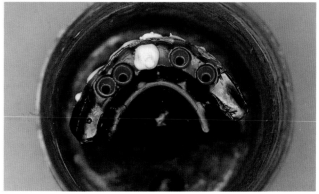

Fig. 9.6

Initial casting process.

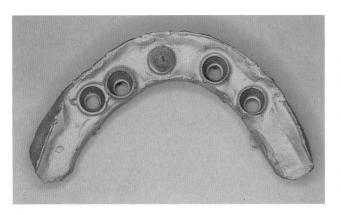
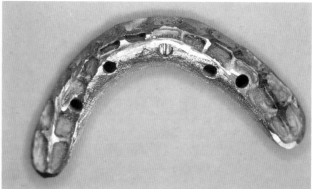

Figs. 9.7 and 9.8

Lower and upper views of cast framework after polishing. The screw in the central gold cylinder can be seen.

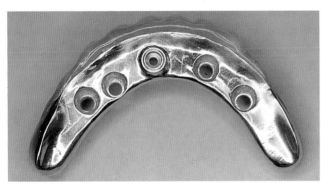
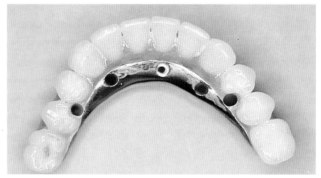

Figs. 9.9 and 9.10

Upper and lower views of the completed prosthesis. It can be seen that only the central cylinder is part of the framework. The rest are chimneys with flat upper bases where the gold cylinders will rest once installed. This has been previously adjusted in the laboratory to avoid soft tissue contact, which can be confirmed with Fit-Checker.

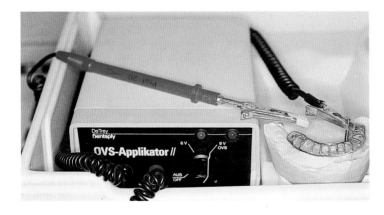

Fig. 9.11

OVS-Applikator device (De Trey) that is used for tin-plating the inner surfaces of the chimneys and external surfaces of the gold cylinders.

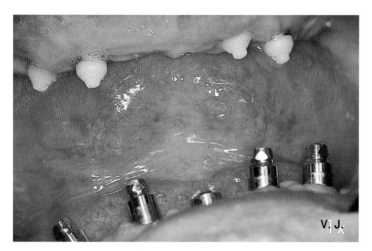

Fig. 9.12

The cylinders are fixed in the mouth to their corresponding standard abutments, except for the central, which is incorporated in the prosthesis.

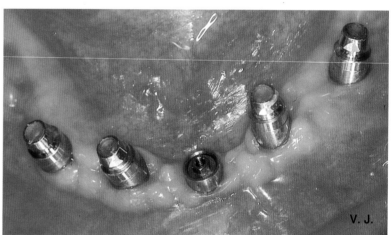

Fig. 9.13

The screw-access holes are blocked out with wax so that the resin does not flow into them during cementing.

Fig. 9.14

The lingual accesses to the caps are blocked out in the hybrid prosthesis. The gold cylinders will be cemented to the caps afterward.

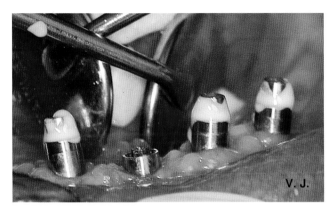
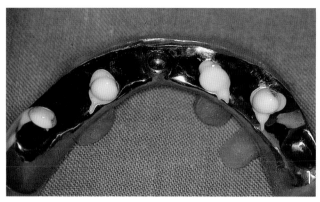

Figs. 9.15 and 9.16

Panavia is placed around the gold cylinders in the mouth. The area has to be very dry, so the assistant must keep the tongue away by using two retractors. Using the same material, we fill the prosthesis caps, making sure we do not trap air bubbles.

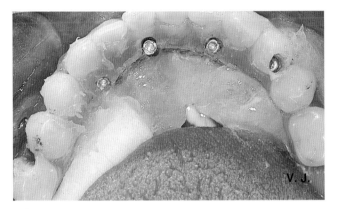
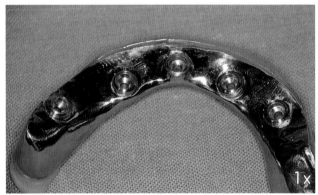

Fig. 9.17

The prosthesis is now placed over the abutments, with care taken to tighten sufficiently the screw of the central gold cylinder, which is included in the framework, so that it all fits perfectly in place.

The wax is quickly removed from the prosthesis and entranceway to the gold cylinders, so as to have good access once the anaerobic resin has polymerized.

In the picture it can be seen how the entranceways are open. The rest is covered with petroleum jelly to create an anaerobic environment for the resin to harden.

All excess must be removed previously with a brush.

Allow 10 minutes before unscrewing the prosthesis.

Fig. 9.18

Lower view of the prosthesis just removed from the mouth. Some resin may remain along the periphery if care has not been taken when tin-plating.

This technique can be done in a single phase, cementing all the gold cylinders at once or separately, depending on the difficulty of the case and patient cooperation.

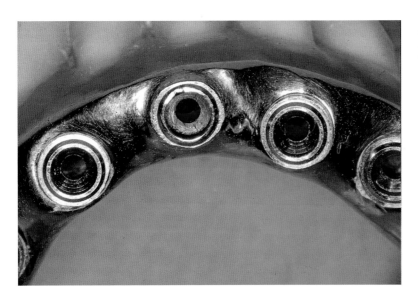

Fig. 9.19

Polished prosthesis.

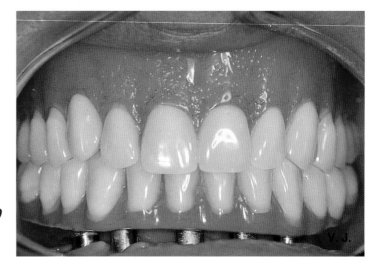

Fig. 9.20

Case completed and installed. Upper overdenture is supported by four implants and the lower is supported by five.

At this time the case is remounted on the articulator to readjust occlusion, if necessary, or this is done directly in the mouth. We are now sure that the prosthesis is going to have an absolutely passive fit on the implants.

Long-term prognosis will be much better.

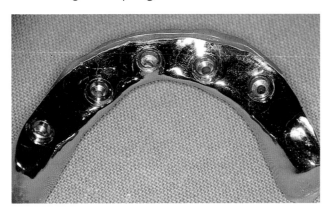

Fig. 9.21

One-year follow-up of the prosthesis.

Contrary to what we would imagine, the area that retained more plaque was the central cylinder, in other words, the one that was overcasted.

The other four were not processed in any way at the laboratory and are in a purer state. When the five standard abutments were checked, they were all found to be perfect.

9.2 Cemented passive-fit conversion of a conventional implant-supported partial prosthesis

We are dealing with a partial prosthesis. Even though the prosthesis had a perfect fit on the cast, it was noticed that while placing and tightening the screws the patient felt a "pulling on the implant." The bothersome overload did not disappear, despite repeated efforts in checking the occlusion. A week later, we decided to redo the case with a new technique based on what was described previously. The gold cylinders were eliminated from the prosthesis, leaving the chimneys, and new cylinders were adapted in the laboratory cast, followed by cementation in the mouth without any need to rebuild the prosthesis.

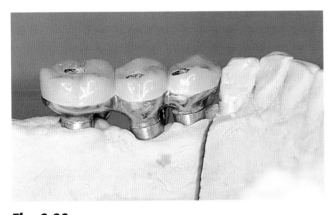

Fig. 9.22

Initial prosthesis on the cast, where on inspection no adjustment difficulties were detected.

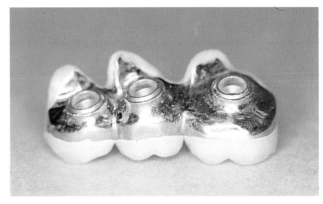

Fig. 9.23

"Apparent contours" were created and the cylinders were overcasted to the framework using standard procedures.

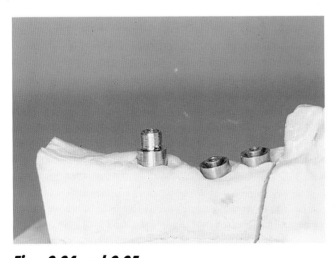

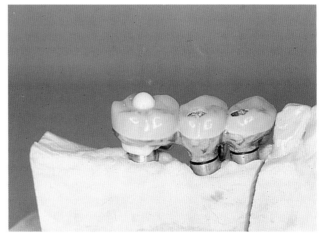

Figs. 9.24 and 9.25

Once the distal cylinder has been removed, a modified one is placed on the cast, checking friction with Fit-Checker.

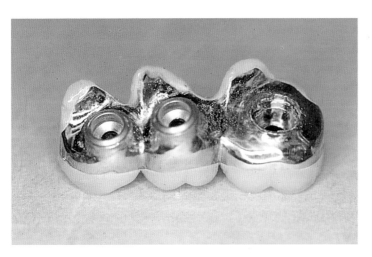

Fig. 9.26

Bottom view of the prosthesis framework once the distal gold cylinder has been eliminated and a chimney or hollowed-out area has been created.

If the existing space between the new chimney and the modified cylinder is too large, it could be waxed up and overcasted. This would minimize the space between both, which is necessary for a good cementing technique.

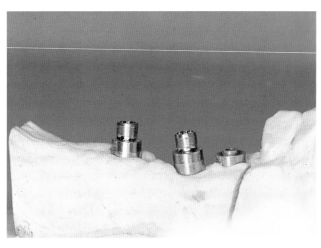
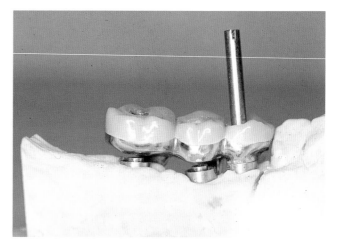

Figs. 9.27 and 9.28

The next step is to modify the second cylinder on the cast, creating a chimney in the prosthesis.

Notice that the mesial cylinder is left untouched because we are certain it will fit 100% once it is installed in the mouth and the contact point is checked.

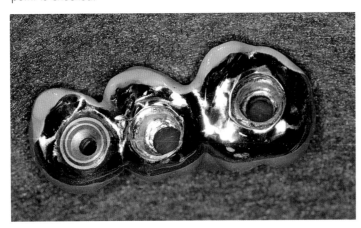

Fig. 9.29

Bottom view of the "modified prosthesis," in which are shown the cylinder and the entrances to the two chimneys, which afterward will be cemented to the two gold cylinders directly in the mouth. Notice that the inner surface has been tin-plated.

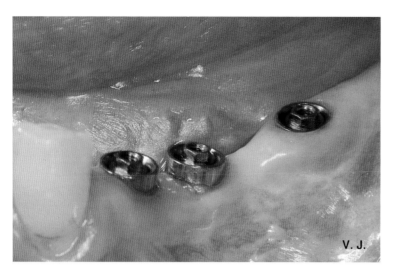

Fig. 9.30

View of the three standard abutments, which are slightly lingualized, forcing us to use the technique of "apparent contours."

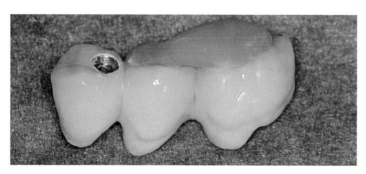

Fig. 9.31

The two distal chimneys are blocked with soft wax.

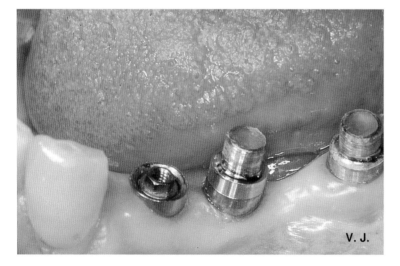

Fig. 9.32

The "modified" tin-plated gold cylinders are installed. The screws are protected with soft wax.

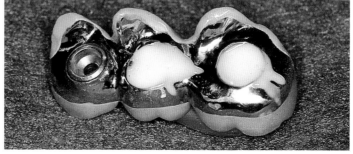

Fig. 9.33

Panavia is placed in the chimneys and also in the cylinders during installation. The prosthesis is screwed to the mesial abutment.

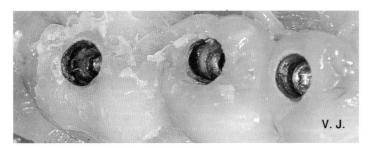

Fig. 9.34

The wax is quickly removed with an excavator and the excess material is removed with a small brush.

Later the air is closed out using petroleum jelly, so that the anaerobic resin hardens. Wait 10 minutes.

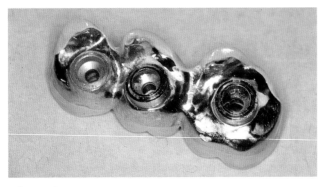

Fig. 9.35

Bottom view of the prosthesis unscrewed and just removed from the mouth.

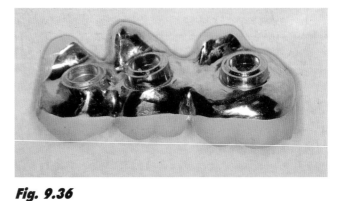

Fig. 9.36

The excess material stuck to the outside is removed and then polished. Notice the big difference in purity between the gold cylinders not overcasted (central and distal) and the mesial that has undergone laboratory procedures.

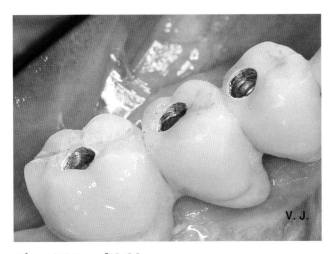

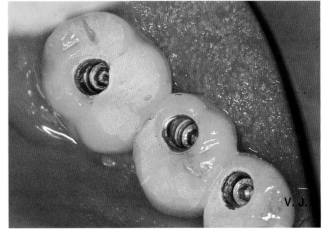

Figs. 9.37 and 9.38

When the prosthesis was installed again, we were surprised to detect that the occlusion had varied; it had to be readjusted in depth. This indicates that there was an undetected error. The "bothersome feeling" immediately disappeared.

In partial prostheses, we believe that the technique of "cemented cylinders over screw-retained prostheses" may be the only way to be certain that we have full passive fit. Who has not had a patient complain of a slight "feeling of pressure" when tightening the prosthesis? Usually it disappears inmediately, but....

In straight frameworks, as in partial prostheses, it is easier to have a good cast with a good fit, as compared to curved frameworks.

In the future, it may be possible that all partial prostheses will be "cemented on screwheld prostheses."

Perhaps the reader is wondering why we do not use techniques that cement the prostheses directly to the implant abutments, thus avoiding possible discrepancies.

The answer is simple. It would be wonderful to have large restorations in fixed prosthodontics over natural dentition always cemented temporarily; this way we could solve future problems like porcelain fractures. This is not feasible, however, because the temporary cement loosens and is washed out. This is why the techniques here described should employ a definitive cement that is very resistant.

With the technique of "screw-type bridges" we always have "temporary cement." If the occlusion is good, with a good fit established with new hexagonal screws and a contra-angle screwdriver, it will never loosen.

On the other hand, it will be possible to introduce variations should natural teeth be lost or porcelain fractures occur, avoiding refabrication of the prosthesis.

9.3 Implant fracture solution using the same prosthesis

Implants can fracture, on occasion, due to adjustment, occlusal parafunction, or design problems. In the following case, the fracture was due to a combination of these factors.

The patient experienced "slight gum pain" in one of the abutments. The prosthesis was removed and the following situation was observed.

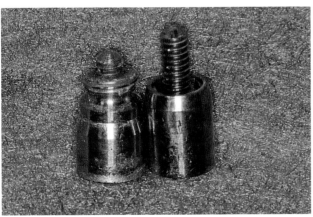

Fig. 9.39

Standard abutment screwed to the fractured implant. The picture compares it to a normal one, but of different size.

For these cases, special accessories are available to smooth the remaining implant surface in the mouth, enabling us to place in another abutment.

Naturally, there will be a slight variation in the insertion axis; thus the cylinder will not fit on the new abutment.

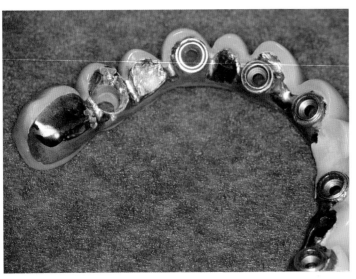

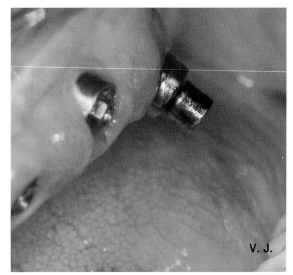

V. J.

Figs. 9.40 and 9.41

Prosthesis ready to have cylinder cemented. This has been modified and adjusted in the mouth by coating it with ink and eliminating the friction spots that appear in the chimney.

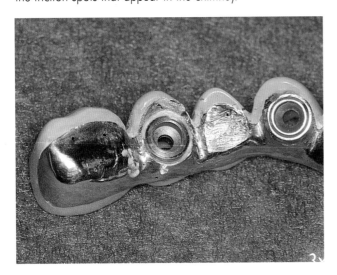

Fig. 9.42

The modified cylinder has been cemented to the prosthesis in the mouth.

The patient initially can wear this without risks until the new one is constructed. This bypasses the use of the unwanted full denture during repair time.

9.4 Additional information

There are doubts as to whether the analogs in the master model are exact duplicates of the mouth.

How many intermediate steps are carried out before the prosthesis is finally installed? How many errors do we introduce?

In this case, we are going to demonstrate that the master model does not coincide with the situation in the mouth.

All the steps of the system (splinting, impressions, pouring, etc) were carried out with utmost care. However, it was observed that there was a slight discrepancy between the master cast and the mouth.

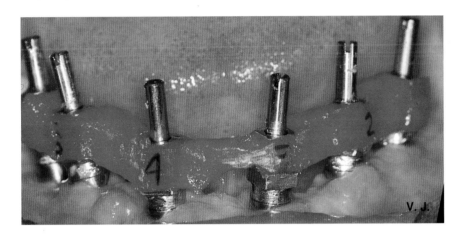

Fig. 9.43

The six abutments are splinted for impression-taking. They are numbered to facilitate their placement in the mouth.

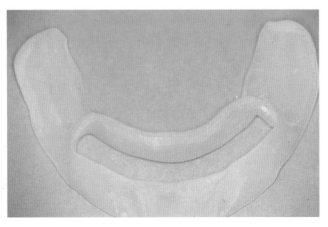 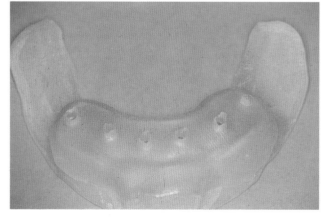

Figs. 9.44 and 9.45

Customized acrylic-resin tray. The window is blocked with soft wax; once placed in the mouth, we check for the correct height of the screws to make sure they can exit.

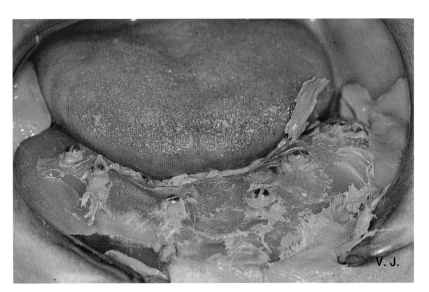

Figs. 9.46 and 9.47

The impression is in the mouth and the screws can be seen surfacing through the wax. These are unscrewed with a "special manual contra-angle" that has special accessories for each case and allows rotational movements in both directions.

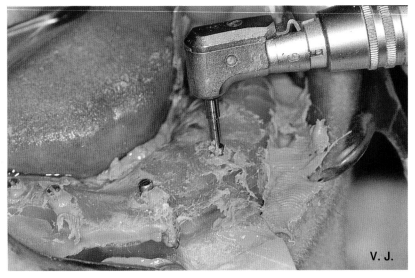

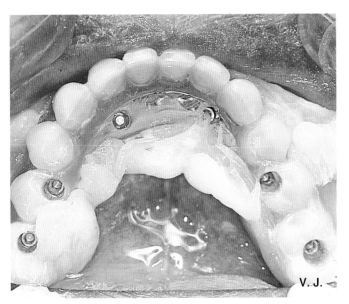

Fig. 9.48

Case being cemented. We have removed the wax and isolated the cement with petroleum jelly.

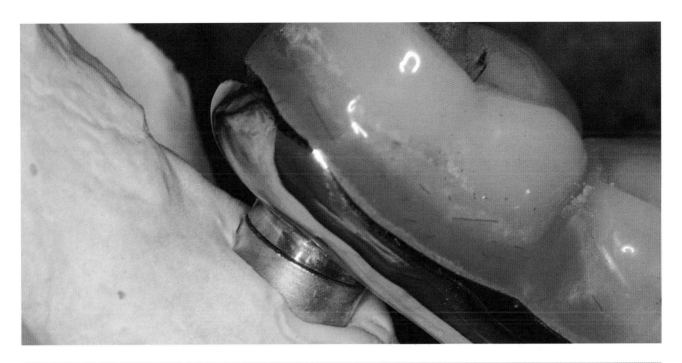

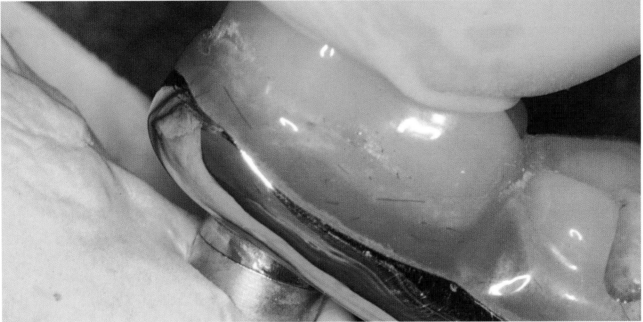

Figs. 9.49 and 9.50

The hybrid prosthesis is placed on the master cast. Passive fit is absent, as seen in the slight misfit in the distal abutment. If we force it manually, we can make it look like it is adjusted, but what about traction forces?

We would not have noticed this in the mouth, and passive fit would still be absent.

In other words, the cast did not match 100% with the real situation.

9.5 Partial prostheses and the cemented coping technique

This technique is quite interesting, because it achieves a perfect passive fit.

The mesial cylinder is not cemented because normally its access is easiest in the mouth.

Case 1

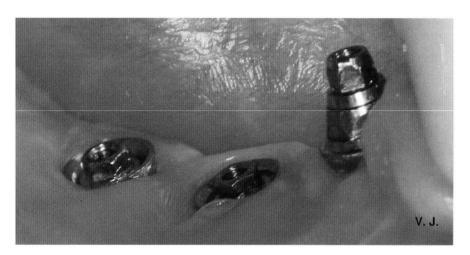

Fig. 9.51

A three-unit prosthesis will be constructed. The most mesial implant has a tapered abutment, while the central and distal abutments are standard.

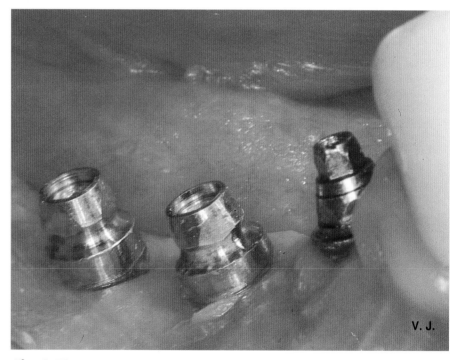

Fig. 9.52

The specific gold cylinders are screwed to the standard abutments. Later, the upper entranceway will be blocked with soft wax to avoid having excess anaerobic resin flow there.

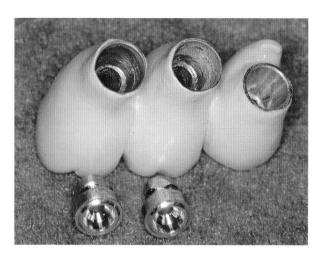

Fig. 9.53

The prosthesis has two chimneys ready to be cemented over the gold cylinders. The most anterior one has a specific gold cylinder for tapered abutments. Here we have built an apparent contour.

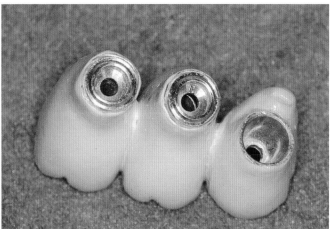

Fig. 9.54

The cylinders have been cemented to the prosthesis.

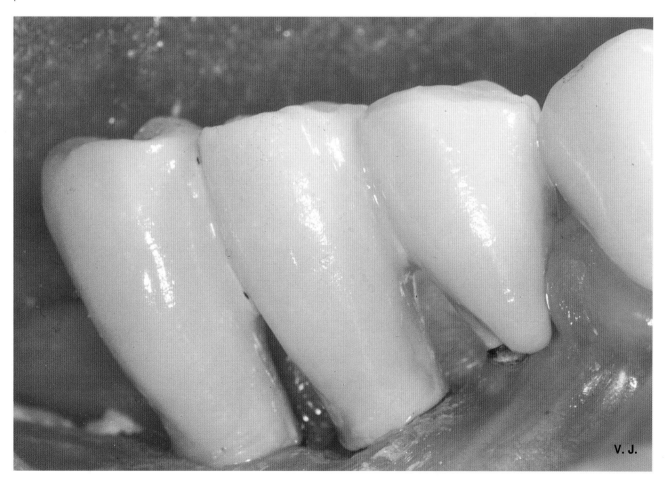

Fig. 9.55

Case completed and installed. Panavia flash is still noticeable, and the wide posterior embrasures will help with hygiene in that area.

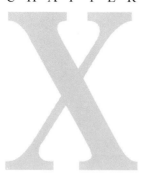

UPPER FIXED RESTORATION

10.1 Technique of the acrylic-resin base with gold cylinders and prefabricated teeth

A) Description

In upper fixed restorations, achieving esthetics is very difficult, since references for the anterior overbite and the patient's smile line are missing.

These and other aspects like centric relation and vertical dimension were explained in chapter VIII in the section describing patient reference registration through the use of "plastic visor." This is helpful when constructing upper overdentures.

Recently, we have developed a new technique for upper fixed restorations that provides a great deal of information for the technician, thus guaranteeing a better final result.

It consists of an acrylic-resin base that includes gold cylinders as well as a set of prefabricated denture teeth that have been selected according to esthetics and implant positioning.

Afterward, it is sectioned in three parts to avoid casting curved frameworks, relating them with or without attachments.

B) Advantages

- Allows for mouth check of cylinder fit on the abutments.

X

- Provides esthetics reference, since in situ framework verification will be similar to that of the final prosthesis.

- Enables us, by adding or removing acrylic resin, to change anterior esthetics by modifying length and shape.

- Creates mouth disoccluding guidances (by adding or removing acrylic resin) and permits us to check and see if centric relation coincides with maximum intercuspation (if this doesn't occur, occlusion should be adjusted until it is achieved).

- Allows the same occlusion to be obtained afterward on the articulator by creating an acrylic-resin index on its incisal table, thus producing a customized anterior guidance.

- Permits the shape to be modified with wax in the laboratory so that once it is evenly reduced and casted, a good occlusion can be obtained, helping to achieve uniform porcelain thickness. This will eliminate future fracture areas.

- Greatly simplifies laboratory procedures.

- Provides esthetic and functional results that are quite acceptable.

10.2 Clinical cases

A) Case 1. Clinical and laboratory procedure description (see chapter XII, section 3.3A).

Patient with a mild Class III malocclusion and crossbite in whom the goal is to achieve edge-to-edge occlusion.

Eight implants were placed, two of which are located in the pterygoid process.

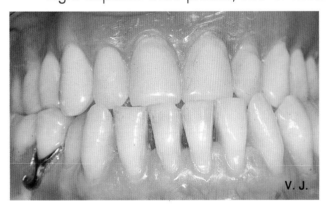 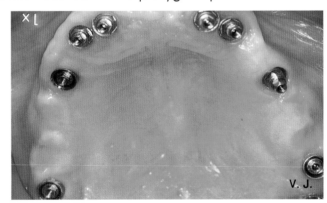

Figs. 10.1 and 10.2

Implants in the mouth, palatal view and initial occlusion with the provisional full denture.

Notice that standard abutments are used in the anterior, while tapered or standard abutments are used in others areas depending on their arch position.

The most distal abutments are located in the pterygoid process and are standard type, because of decreased interarch distance and difficulty in posterior hygiene, and because they are easier to handle in the mouth.

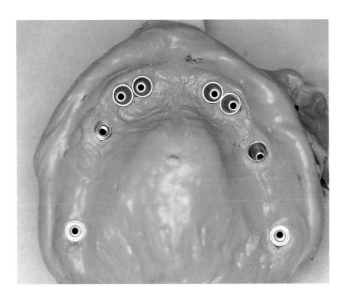

Fig. 10.3

Upper arch impression.

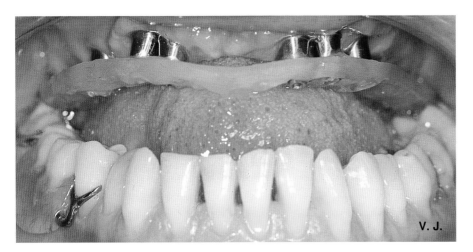

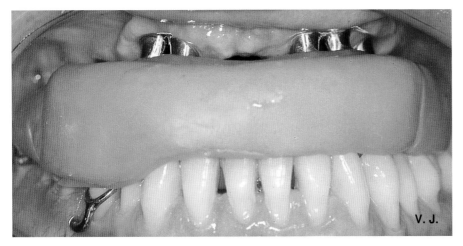

Figs. 10.4 and 10.5

After pouring the impression, the laboratory constructs an acrylic-resin "bite plate" with the gold cylinders enclosed.

The fit enables us to verify that the impression was valid.

Vertical dimension is determined through the usual technique. The posterior acrylic resin had to be reduced because of excessive contact until we reached the patient's exact vertical dimension.

Centric relation is registered using Moyco wax, keeping the posterior area free to check contacts.

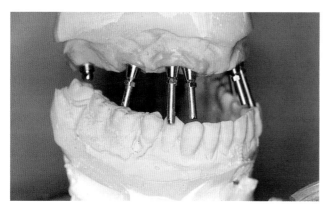

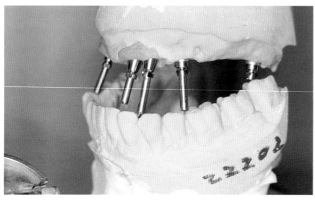

Figs. 10.6 and 10.7

Case mounted on the articulator (right and left lateral view).

The screws exit in good direction. Notice what little space is available in the distal cylinder. Since we are dealing with a third molar, it will be extracted later.

While pouring the impression, soft gingiva was used in the areas related to the tapered cylinders (subgingival shoulder).

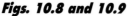

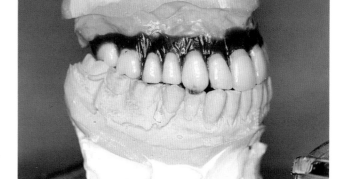

Figs. 10.8 and 10.9

The laboratory screws are changed for gold ones, and by using wax we mount the prefabricated acrylic resin teeth, with the appropiate color, shape, esthetics, and occlusion.

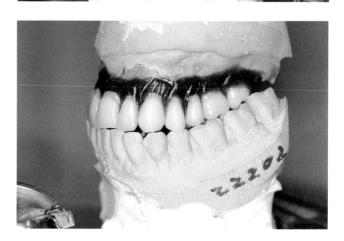

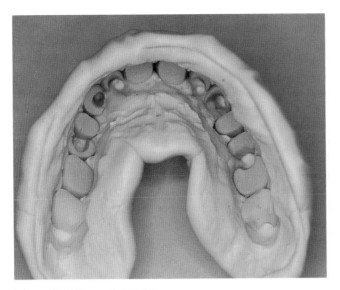

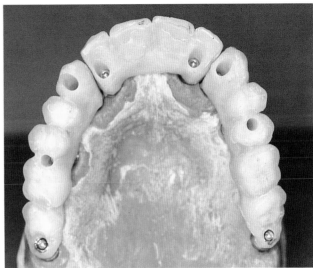

Figs. 10.10 and 10.11

A hard silicone index is taken and it is introduced in hot water to make the wax disappear. Acrylic resin of the same color is then placed in the space created and related to gold cylinder location, allowing it to harden. Once the flash has been trimmed and shaped, the gold cylinders can be seen included in the acrylic structure (see laboratory technique, chapter XII, section 3.3.A).

Notice that the structure has been sectioned into three parts.

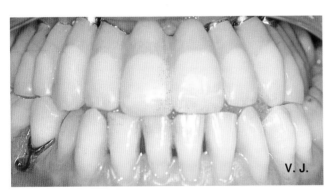

V. J.

Figs. 10.12 and 10.13

The acrylic-resin prostheses are installed, and the fit over the abutments is verified.

In this phase esthetics, shape, color, and smile line are checked.

The occlusion is adjusted to make centric relation coincide with maximum intercuspation.

Acrylic resin is added or removed to determine a guide for anterior disocclusion (see chapter IV, section 2.C).

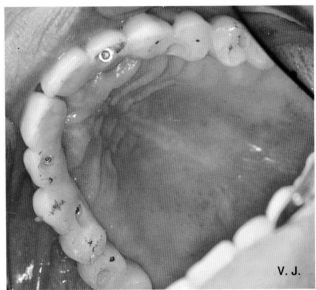

V. J.

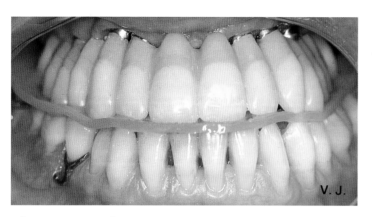

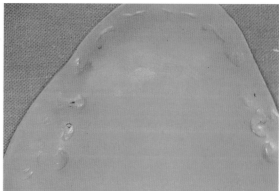

Figs. 10.14 and 10.15

Once the arches are well related, a centric bite wafer is taken to check tooth mounting on the articulator. It can be modified if necessary. Imprint depth on the wafer must be minimal.

Protrusive registrations can be taken and the condylar inclination is adjusted on the articulator. Lateral registrations may also be taken to record the Bennett angle.

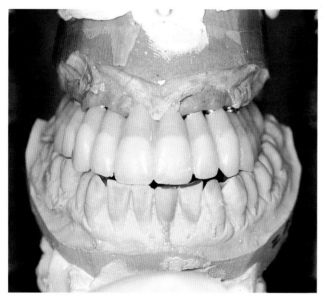

Figs. 10.16 and 10.17

The case is mounted again or simply checked if modifications are not necessary.

On the incisal table of the articulator, the protrusive and lateral guides are recorded with acrylic resin. These were constructed in the mouth.

By using these, porcelain anterior guidance can be constructed.

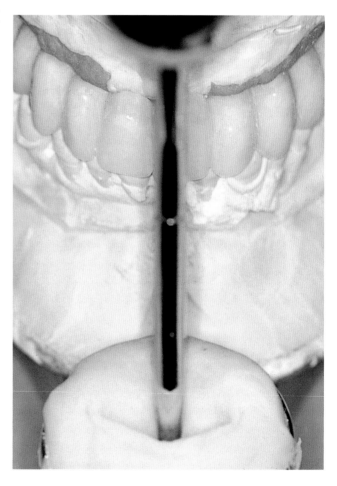

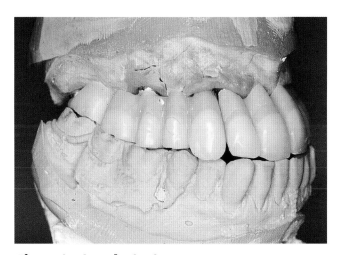

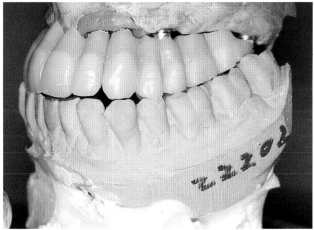

Figs. 10.18 and 10.19

Lateral view. Posterior occlusion can be improved through anatomical carving. At this time it is helpful to contour by adding or removing acrylic resin.

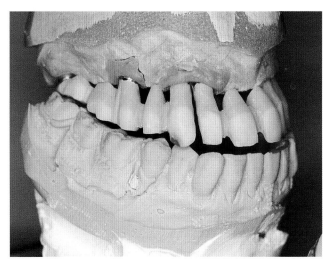

Figs. 10.20 and 10.21

One millimeter of acrylic resin must be reduced evenly for the framework that is to be cast. Observe how posterior anatomy has changed.

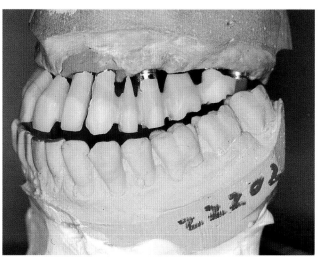

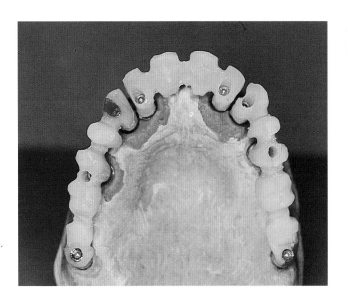

Fig. 10.22

Palatal view of the whole framework.

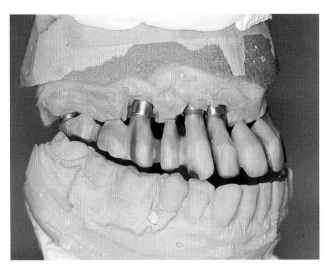 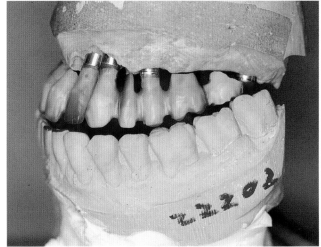

Figs. 10.23 and 10.24

The areas to be recontoured or where interproximal contact needs refining can be waxed up. Once this is finished, it is ready to be cast.

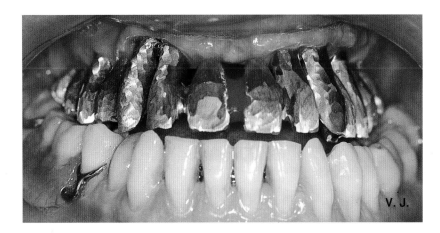

Fig. 10.25

Once cast and polished, it is installed for verification.

Notice that the anterior (curved surface) had to be sectioned and splinted with Duralay because of lack of fit.

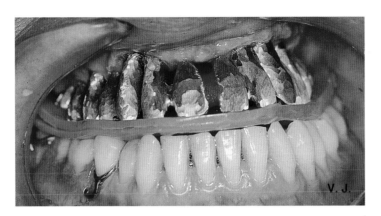

Fig. 10.26

A new wax registration is taken to reverify the new arrangement on the articulator. This is done in case the previous checks were not satisfactory.

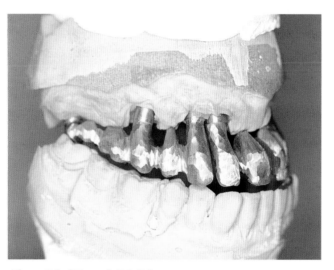

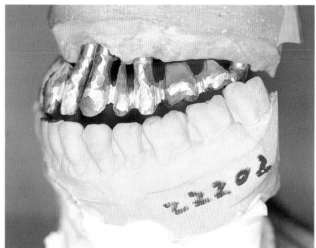

Figs. 10.27 and 10.28

Lateral view of the framework before anterior soldering.

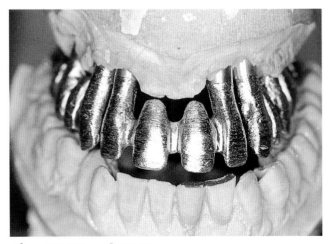

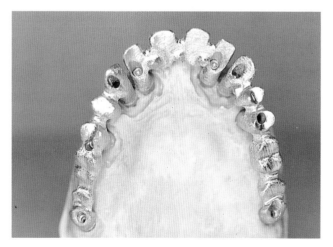

Figs. 10.29 and 10.30

The anterior segment has been soldered (buccal and lingual views).

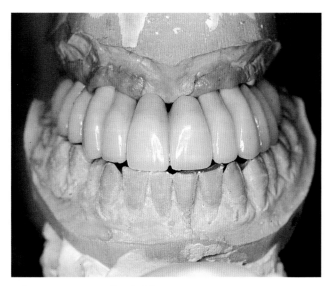
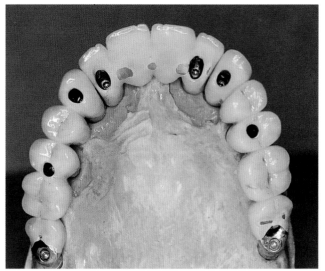

Figs. 10.31 and 10.32

Porcelain prosthesis completed (buccal and palatal views).

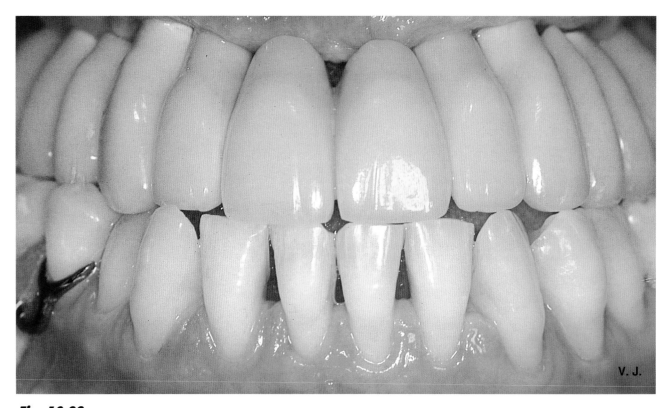

Fig. 10.33

Once the prosthesis is installed, the occlusion, fit, interproximal brush hygiene, and gingival compression should be checked again.

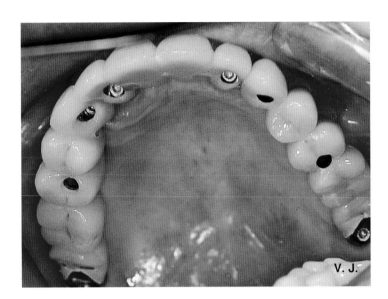

Fig. 10.34

Lingual view of the case.

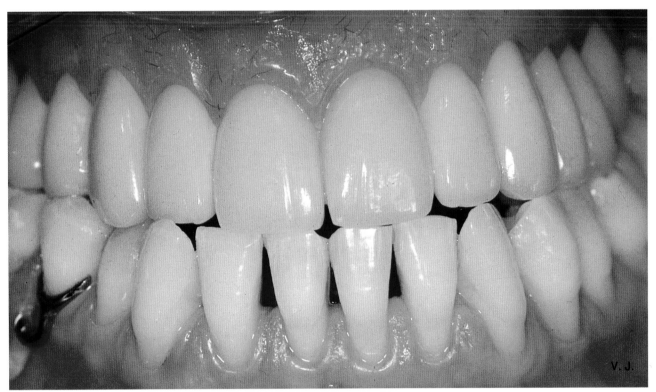

Fig. 10.35

While smiling, the teeth were too obvious, so it was mutually decided to place artificial cosmetic gingiva without attachments to give upper lip support. Consequently, esthetics were enhanced.

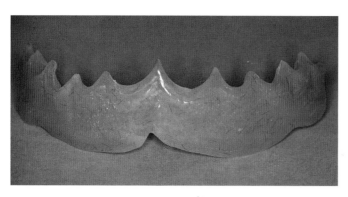

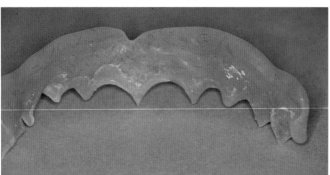

Figs. 10.36 and 10.37

Anterior and posterior views of the rigid artificial gingiva without attachments.

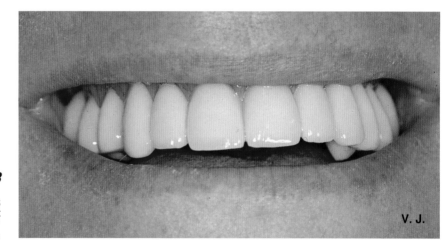

V. J.

Fig. 10.38

Patient's smile shows good esthetics achieved through the use of artificial gingiva.

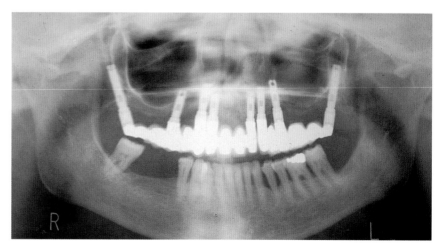

R   L

Fig. 10.39

Panoramic radiograph of the completed case, in which perfect fit over the abutments can be seen.

B) Case 2. Additional information on the same technique but in a different case.

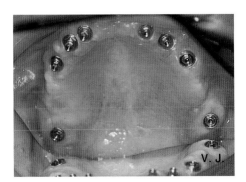

Fig. 10.40

Case presentation. There is favorable anterior implant positioning due to increased implant separation.

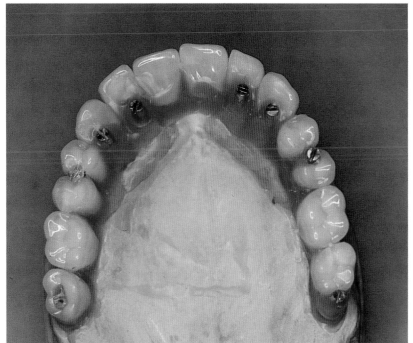

Figs. 10.41 and 10.42

Palatal view of teeth mounted in wax and in acrylic resin after the silicone index and relining were performed. The excess should be eliminated.

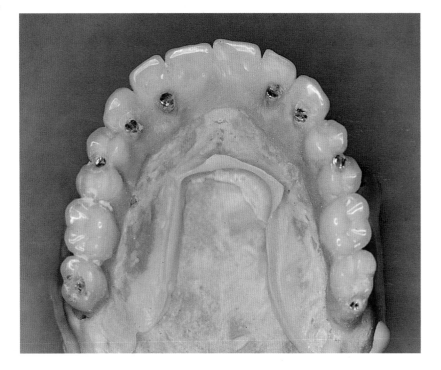

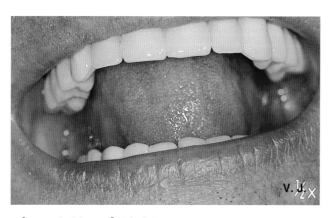
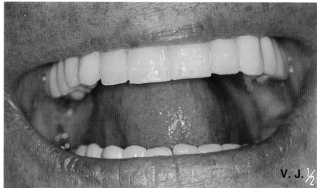

Figs. 10.43 and 10.44

Anterior tooth length has been modified in the acrylic-resin try-in to improve esthetics.

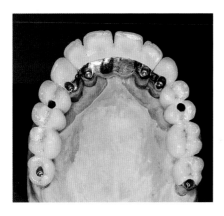

Figs. 10.45 and 10.46

Good implant position allowed for a straighter anterior framework, which was joined to the others through two Plasta attachments (Cendres et Metaux).

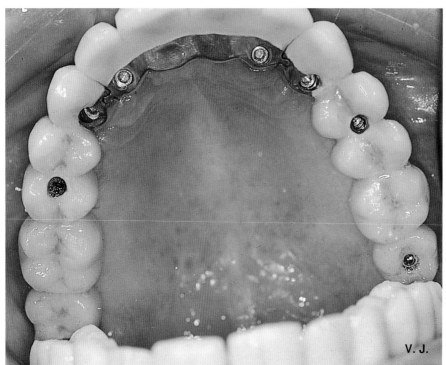

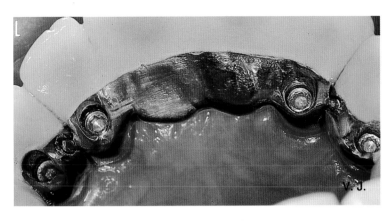

Fig. 10.47

Palatal close-up view of the anterior.

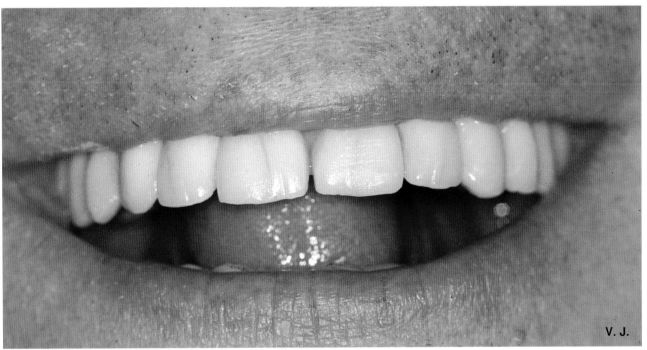

Fig. 10.48

Forced smile in completed case.

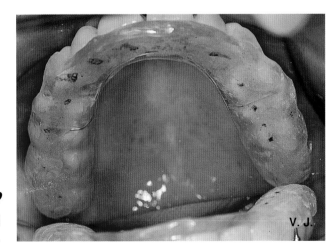

Fig. 10.49

Due to bruxism, an occlusal nightguard
had to be used for protection.

C) Case 3. Technique summary.

For better understanding, an outline-form summary is described on the different framework options available with this technique.

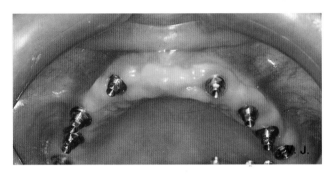

Fig. 10.50

Installed implants. The adequate positioning allowed for tapered abutments, except for the two distal ones.

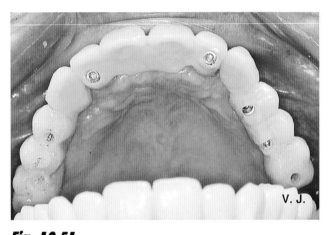

Fig. 10.51

Try-in of the acrylic-resin base with gold cylinders and prefabricated teeth.

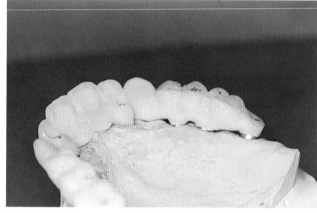

Fig. 10.52

Acrylic structure mounted on the cast.

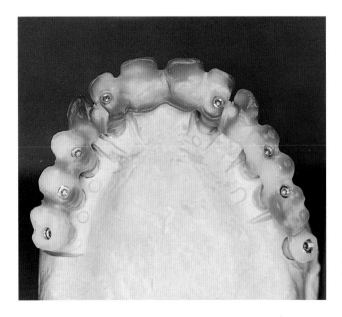

Fig. 10.53

Even recontouring of the acrylic structure, adding wax to those areas where reinforcement of improved anatomy is needed. At this time, two attachments are placed distal to the lateral incisor. This will splint the framework and take into account future implant failure, which can later be solved by soldering.

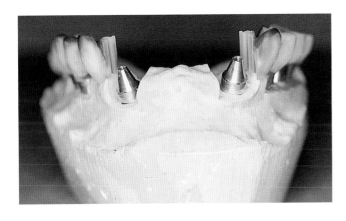

Fig. 10.54

Anterior view of the attachments once the anterior segment has been removed from the cast. Notice the straight design of the posterior framework.

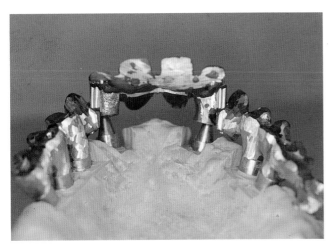
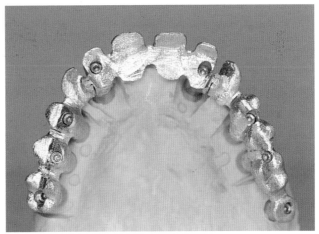

Figs. 10.55 and 10.56

Cast framework. It consists of three straight segments locked to each other to form a single unit.

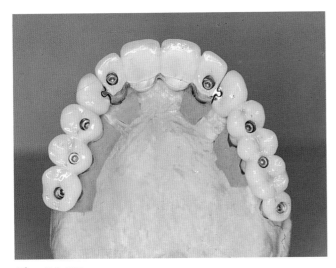
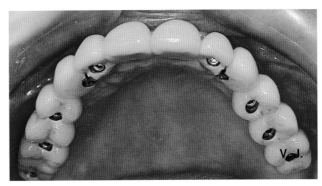

Fig. 10.58

Prosthesis installed.

Fig. 10.57

Once the porcelain is placed, the prosthesis is completed.

10.3 Upper anterior restoration without implants

Another solution to obtain good anterior esthetics is to place the implants distal to the canines.

It is important that the patient is not a clencher and that enough bone is available in the maxillary sinus to place long implants, because of possible overloads in that sector.

On the other hand, the alveolar ridge should be adequate to achieve good esthetics.

The following case is courtesy of Dr. José Manuel Navarro Alonso.

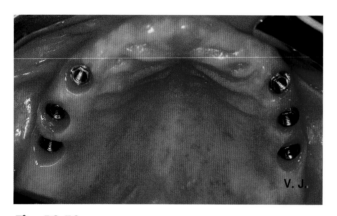

Fig. 10.59

Six maxillary implants were placed, leaving the anterior segment untouched.

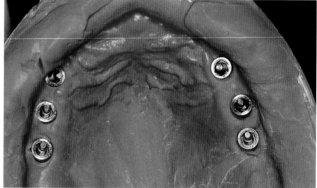

Fig. 10.60

In the impression, UCLA abutments were used. These were the abutments employed to treat this case.

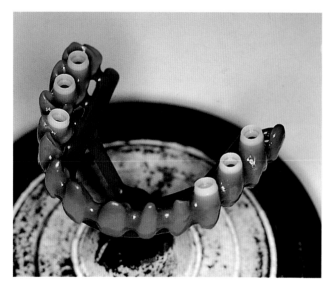

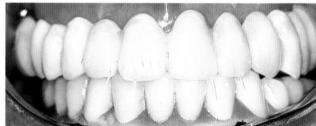

Fig. 10.62

Final prosthesis installed.

Fig. 10.61

Waxup ready for casting.

10.4 Combined cemented-cylinder technique: angulated abutments

This case was treated for the first time in 1988, when angulated abutments were not available. All treatment modalities used and the errors in treatment shall be discussed. Emphasis will be placed on the maxillary treatment.

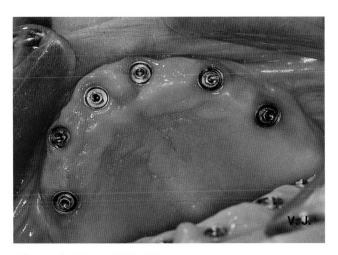 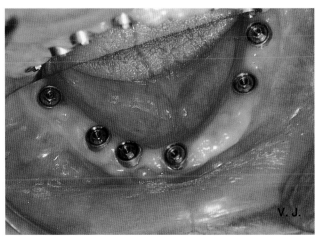

Figs. 10.63 and 10.64

Patient with six upper and six lower implants.

The mandible was treated first, relating it to the upper full denture. Two months later, the maxilla was treated.

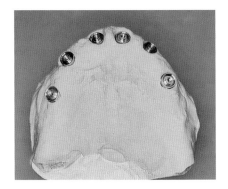 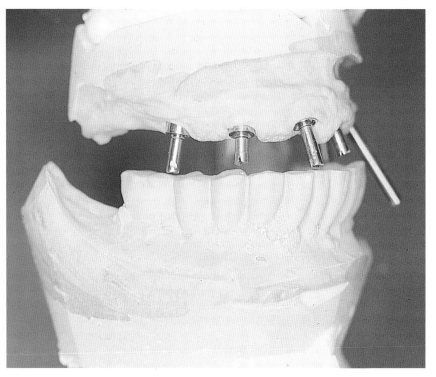

Figs. 10.65 and 10.66

Upper cast mounted on the articulator. Notice that the direction of the left upper canine implant is toward the buccal.

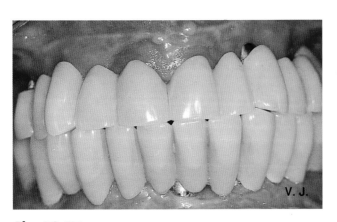

Fig. 10.67

An upper acrylic-resin prosthesis was constructed, with poor canine esthetics.

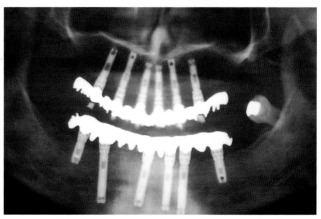

Fig. 10.68

Radiograph upon completion of the case.

The upper left canine was fragile; consequently, a fracture occurred a year later. The prosthesis had to be reconstructed, so it was decided to redesign it in order to achieve thicker acrylic-resin surface and resistance.

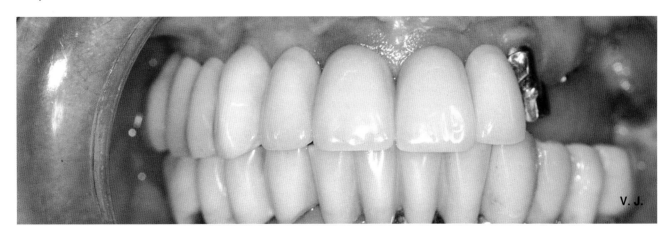

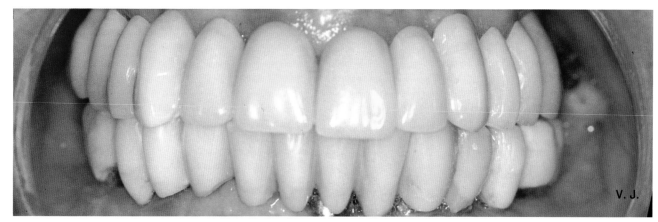

Figs. 10.69 and 10.70

An overstructure was prepared by constructing the prosthesis in two parts.

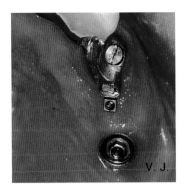

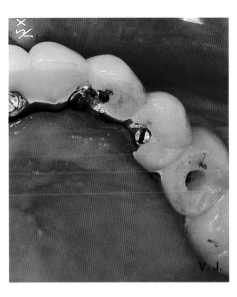

Figs. 10.71 and 10.72

The canine was milled with an additional screw hole in the cantilever. The overstructure was screw-retained on this and the most distal implant.

Due to the great leverage introduced in that area, a few years later the patient presented with slight pain around the most distal implant and the gingiva. The prosthesis was removed and we found that the implant had fractured.

The first prosthesis was used as a provisional until the new prosthesis could be constructed, because the patient had lost the full denture. The provisional was readapted using the cemented-cylinder technique to achieve a good fit on the aforementioned implant (see chapter IX, section 9.3).

At this time, angulated abutments were available, which, because of their versatility to change positions, we decided to use to solve the canine esthetic problem.

Combining angulated and tapered abutments can create insertion problems, which can be avoided by placing the angulated abutments with the exact inclination.

The canine implants, inclination made the abutment selection difficult. Consequently, a UCLA-type impression coping was placed directly on the implant.

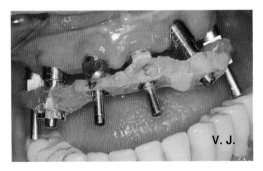

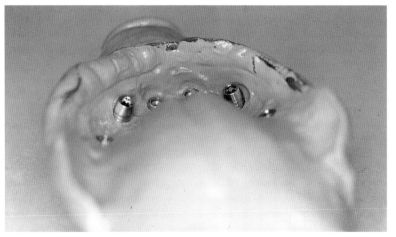

Figs. 10.73 and 10.74

Observe the accessories mentioned previously at the canines with a hexagonal base.

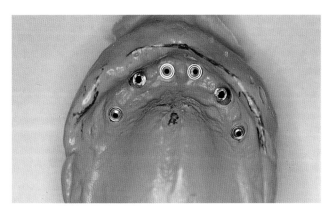

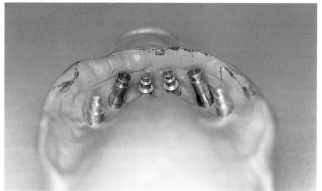

Figs. 10.75 and 10.76

Standard impression copings were used in the four other implants. The analogs are placed in their corresponding copings.

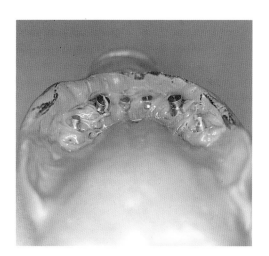

Fig. 10.77

The impression is prepared for a soft gingival model and then poured.

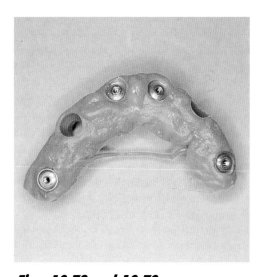

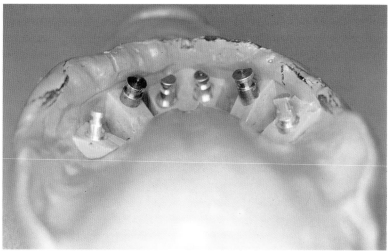

Figs. 10.78 and 10.79

The soft gingiva, once hardened, is removed. It is then sectioned to avoid undercuts. It is placed again and poured.

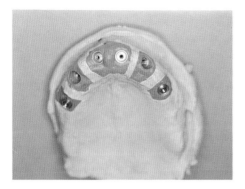

Fig. 10.80

Soft-gingiva cast model. In the canines, the implant analogs can be seen; the rest are the standard abutments.

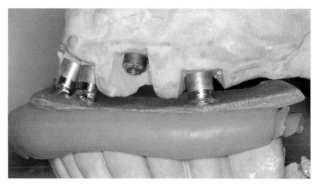

Fig. 10.81

Using the standard copings (four) an acrylic-resin base plate is constructed. Centric relation and vertical dimension are registered in the mouth, to be mounted afterward on the articulator.

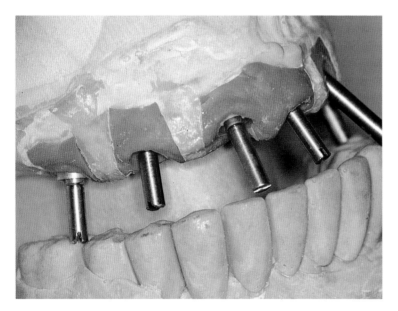

Fig. 10.82

The case study shows that the direction of the upper right canine is adequate for a standard abutment. The upper left canine, however, will need an angulated abutment. Notice the change in screw direction that occurs.

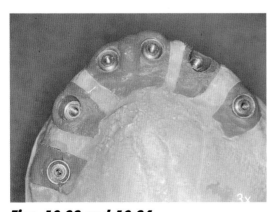
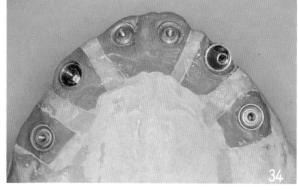

Figs. 10.83 and 10.84

Screw-retained standard and angulated abutments over the implant analog (before and after).

Now the position of the angulated abutment must be determined, but since the rest are standard abutments there will not be insertion difficulties when installing. If they were to be related with tapered abutments, it would be easier to work on the model instead of the mouth. One of the reasons is that it is simpler to find parallelism with a surveyor.

Once the correct position is determined on the cast model, an accessory that relates this to the mouth is needed.

It occurred to us to adapt the same cylinder to permit the exact entry of both screws of the angulated abutment. This way the same position will be obtained after installation as existed on the model.

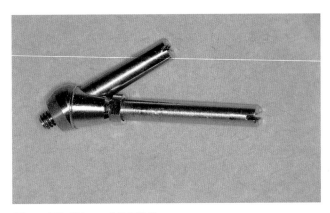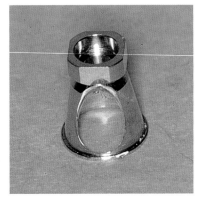

Figs. 10.85 and 10.86
Angulated abutment and the adapted cylinder. A window was opened and a ledge was milled to allow the entry and perfect fit of the screws.

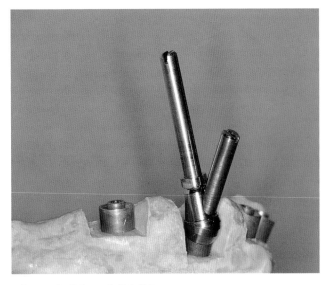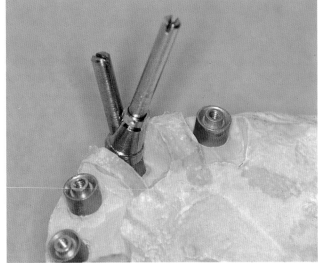

Figs. 10.87 and 10.88
The angulated abutment is screwed to the implant analog through the use of a short screw. The adapted gold cylinder is fixed to the angulated abutment with a long screw. Anterior and posterior views.

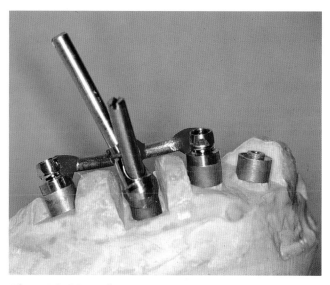

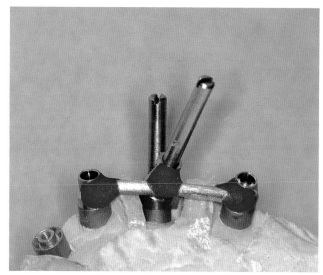

Figs. 10.89 and 10.90

The gold cylinders are placed in the corresponding adjacent standard abutments and splinted to the angulated one with acrylic resin (Duralay).

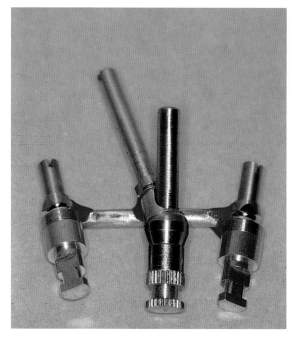

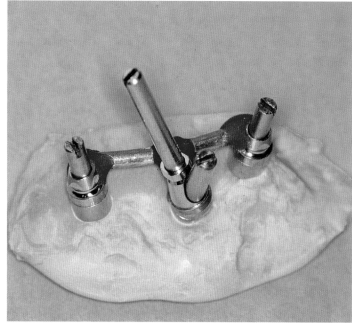

Figs. 10.91 and 10.92

The assembly is removed from the cast model and the analogs are placed. Before investing and soldering, they are incorporated into a plaster base.

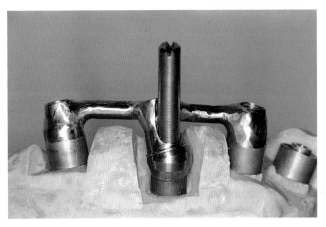
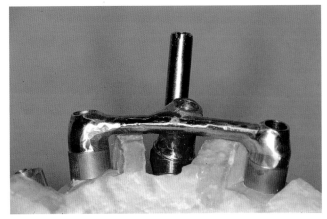

Figs. 10.93 and 10.94

Fixed structure on the working cast. Three gold cylinders joined by a bar can be seen here. While placing a single screw, the fit is verified. The soldering has been completed.

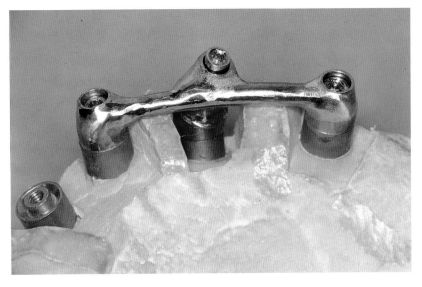

Figs. 10.95 and 10.96

The gold screws are placed. Lateral and occlusal views.

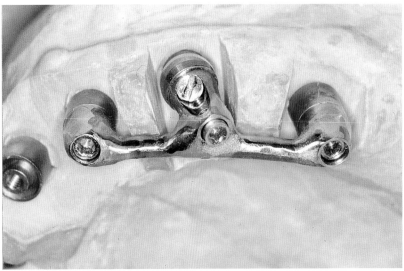

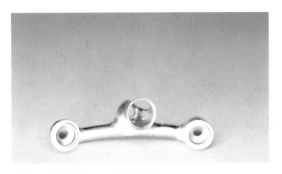
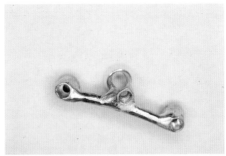

Figs. 10.97 and 10.98

Customized accessory to place the angulated abutment in the mouth. Two standard gold cylinders adapted to the angulated one can be seen here.

The following step is to check its fit in the mouth. The standard abutment over the upper left canine implant is removed, and with the help of the customized accessory the angulated abutment is positioned.

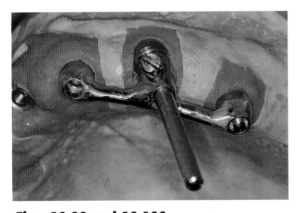
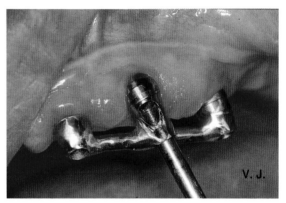

Figs. 10.99 and 10.100

On the cast and placed in the mouth.

Once the fit is checked, the next step is to use the technique of acrylic-resin teeth and gold cylinders, as described in this chapter.

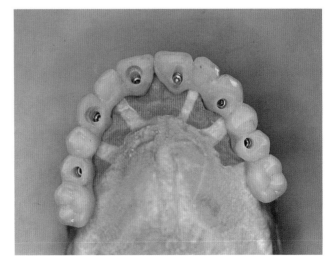

Fig. 10.101

The different gold cylinders included in the acrylic-resin structure.

Since several intermediate steps will be taken, which could vary the final fit in this case, the "cemented-cylinder technique" was preferred to obtain a perfect fit, especially considering that the starting point was a fracture of the upper left distal implant. To do this, the cylinders have to be individualized, creating chimneys and joining them to the acrylic-resin base. This will be done to the four distal implants; the two central ones will remain included in the framework.

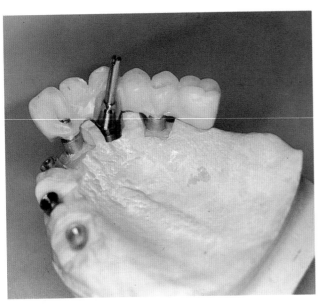

Fig 10.102

Gold cylinder preparation.

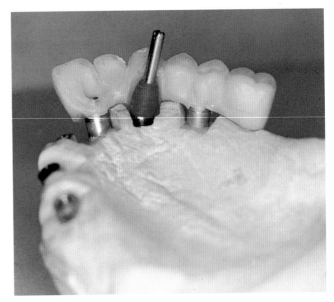

Fig. 10.103

Once the undercuts are blocked out with wax, a chimney is built over the cylinder.

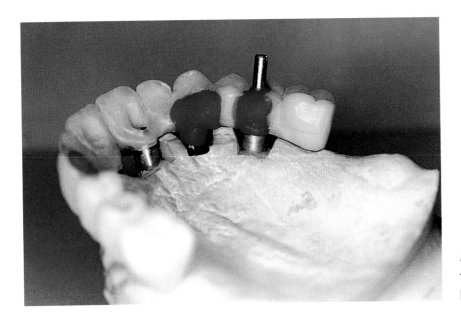

Fig. 10.104

The chimney is joined to the structure with Duralay acrylic resin.

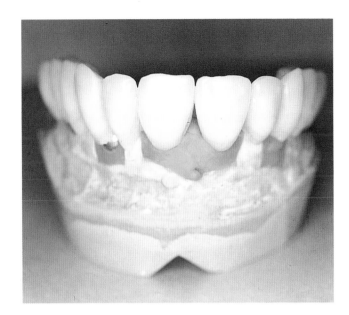

Fig. 10.105

Two independent prostheses, supported by three implants each, can be seen here.

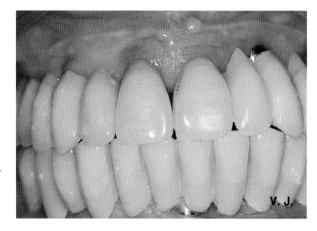

Figs. 10.106 and 10.107

Mouth try-in. At this time, occlusion and esthetics can be modified.

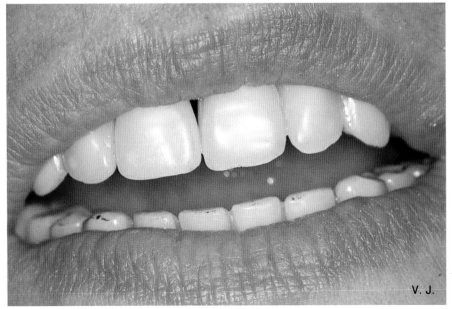

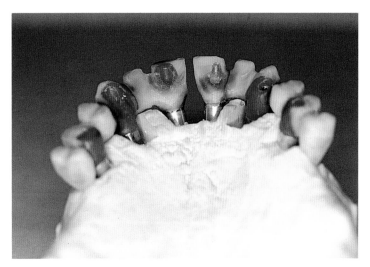

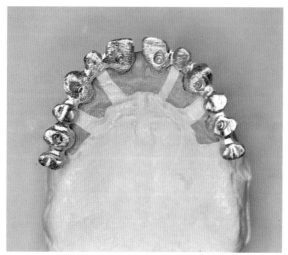

Figs. 10.108 and 10.109
The acrylic resin is reduced evenly, readjusting with wax, and then cast.

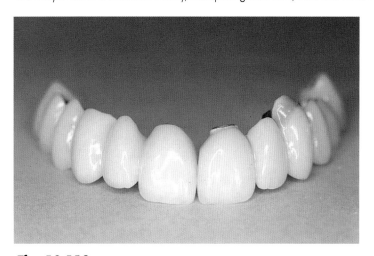

Fig. 10.110
Pink-colored porcelain has been placed on the canine to hide the tooth's excessive length.

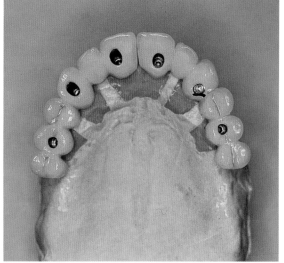

Fig. 10.111
Screw-retained prosthesis over the two central incisors, whose cylinders are within. The other cylinders are fully independent and are placed in the chimneys.

This technique introduces an important esthetic innovation, which is buccal morphology modification with the angled abutment on the cast. This way, important space is gained and position in the mouth will be exactly the same.

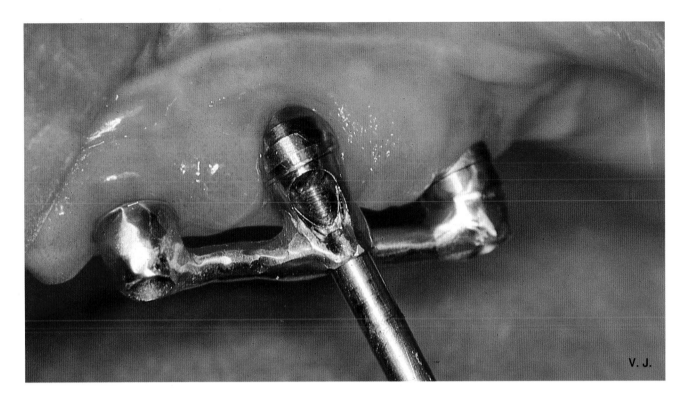

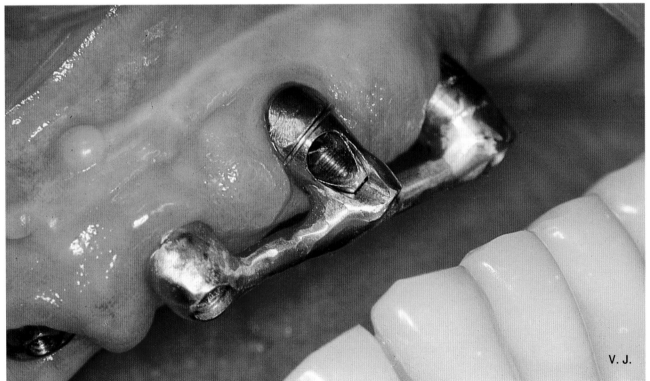

Figs. 10.112 and 10.113

Mouth buccal contour variation before and after cast model correction, which allowed for better esthetics during prosthesis construction. Without the technique, this would have been impossible.

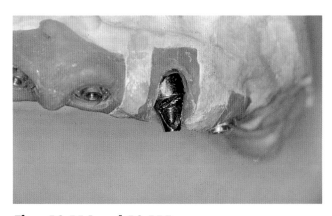
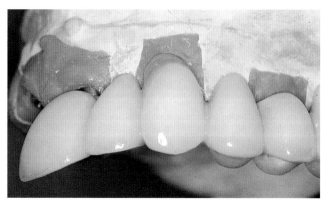

Figs. 10.114 and 10.115

Buccal readaption of the abutment on the model and final result after fit and esthetic adjustment of the prosthesis.

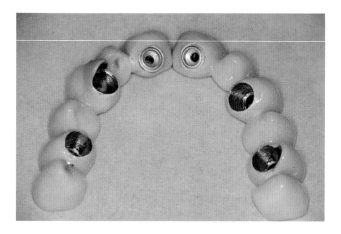

Figs. 10.116 and 10.117

The following step is to cement it in the mouth. Notice the chimneys and how the angulated abutment and the gold cylinders are positioned.

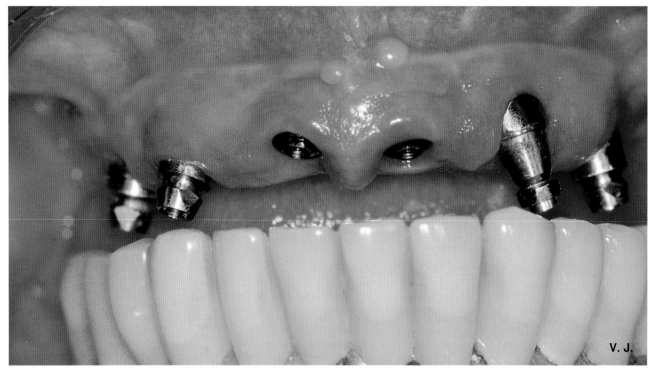

V. J.

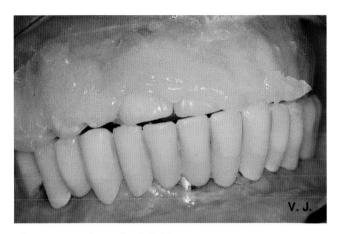
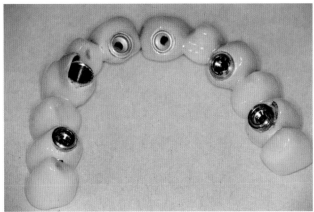

Figs. 10.118 and 10.119

The cemented-cylinder technique requires cement isolation with petroleum jelly for anaerobic resin polymerization. The prosthesis is shown with the cylinder cemented.

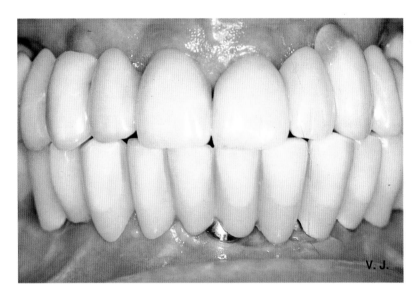

Figs. 10.120 and 10.121

Final result in the mouth. Artificial gingiva was used because the patient preferred the facial esthetics.

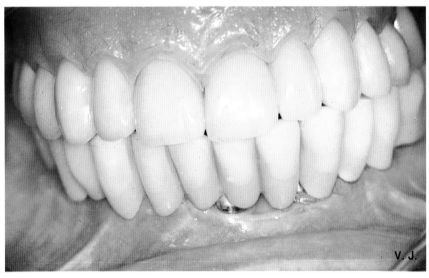

10.5 Use of telescopic crowns as additional support in an upper restoration

Situations sometimes exist in which there are intermediate teeth with adequate periodontium but, because of lack of bone and the prognosis, it is difficult to substitute them for implants, especially in the distal area close to the maxillary sinus.

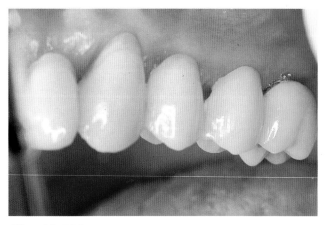

Fig. 10.122

Porcelain-fused-to-metal fixed prosthesis over two implants and two teeth with telescopic crowns (courtesy of Dr. Jaime A. Gil).

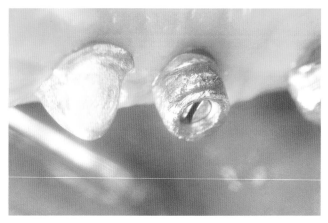

Fig. 10.123

A natural tooth and an osseointegrated implant as fixed-prosthesis anterior abutments.

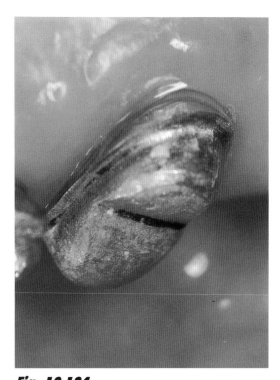

Fig. 10.124

Fixed-prosthesis posterior abutment made up of a cemented coping that serves as an infrastructure for the telescopic crown.

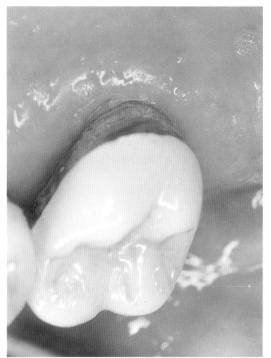

Fig. 10.125

Porcelain-fused-to-metal crown with a telescopic superstructure cemented to the underlying coping.

CHAPTER

XI

PROVISIONAL PROSTHESES

This chapter is very important, because it is necessary to have good provisionals when esthetics are involved or soft tissue healing is needed.

Specific accessories that are now available will be described. In cases using standard and tapered abutments and gold cylinders that can be retrieved and employed again, there is the chance that they can be damaged during handling.

11.1 Specific accessory for CeraOne provisional abutments

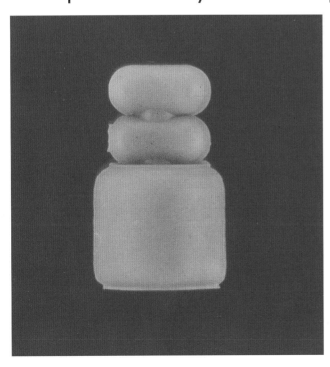

Fig. 11.1

This accessory was described in chapter V, section 5.1.

193

11.2 Specific accessories for provisional standard and tapered abutments

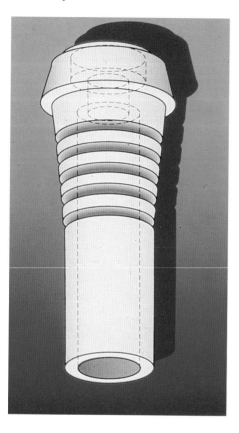

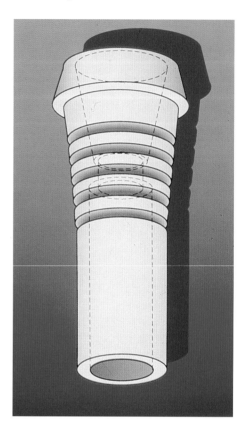

Fig. 11.2

This figure represents the plastic accessory that is screw-retained on the standard abutment. The "female," or matrix, which is included in the temporary prosthesis, fits on the abutment.

Fig. 11.3

The same sheath for use in tapered abutments.

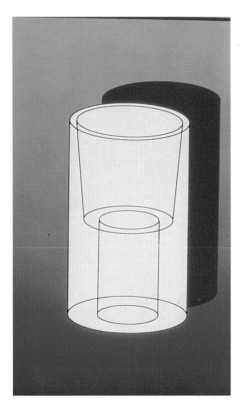

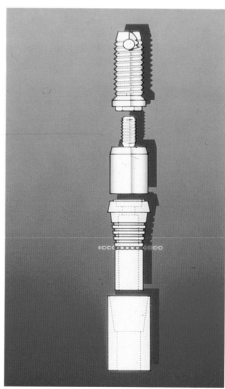

Fig. 11.4

This is the matrix that can be cemented to the male (patrix) or can be friction-retained.

Fig. 11.5

Interrelationship of the aforementioned accessories. From bottom to top there is a matrix, patrix, abutment (standard in this case), and the implant.

11.3 Clinical case: posterior acrylic-resin provisionals

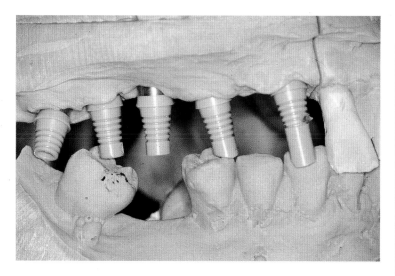

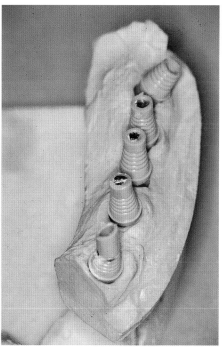

Figs. 11.6 and 11.7

The plastic matrixes, once placed on the cast and depending on the occlusion, have their height adjusted with the opponent. Buccal and occlusal views.

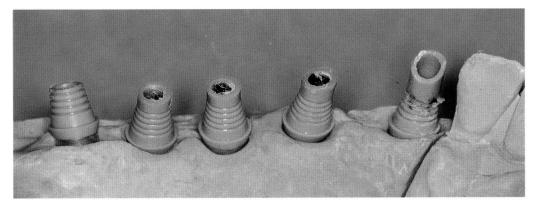

Fig. 11.8

The cast is sectioned for easy laboratory handling. In those implant cases in which no intermediate natural teeth are present, the abutments do not need to be individualized, but must be done in a block, so that the interrelationship between them does not vary. It is important to achieve a precise fit over the different types of abutments (in this case standard and tapered) when installed. Palatal view.

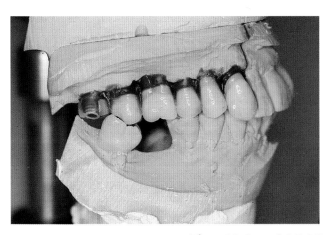

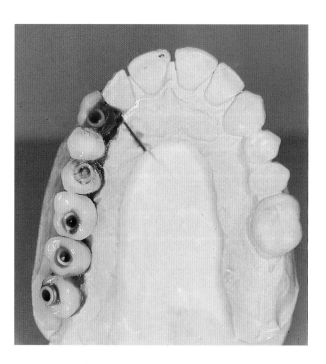

Figs. 11.9 and 11.10

The prefabricated teeth are mounted and adapted with wax. Lateral and occlusal views.

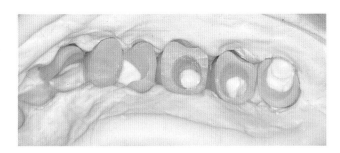

Fig. 11.11

A hard-setting silicone index is taken and the wax is eliminated with hot water.

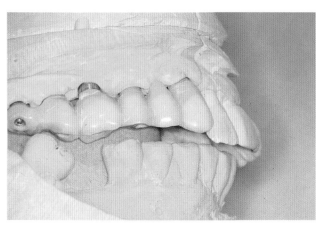

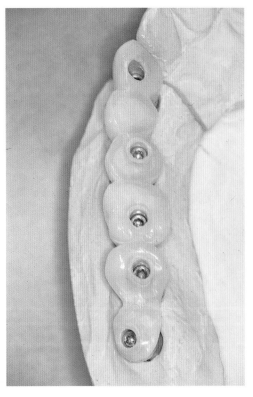

Figs. 11.12 and 11.13

The index with the teeth included is placed again on the cast over the male provisional accessories and then relined with acrylic resin of the same color.

The flash is removed and it is contoured, adjusting it with respect to the gingiva. Lateral and occlusal views after processing and polishing are shown.

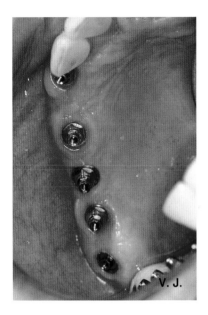

Fig. 11.14

View of installed abutments, showing four tapered and one standard, which is the type preferred for the most distal areas.

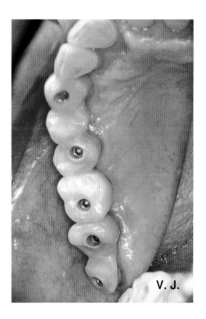

Fig. 11.15

Installed provisional acrylic-resin prosthesis, occlusal view.

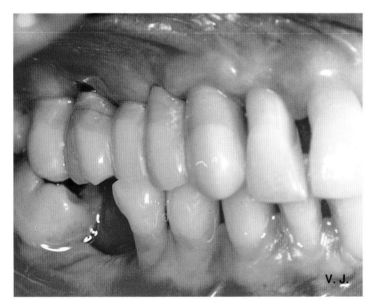

Fig. 11.16

Lateral view: the first-molar standard abutment will have to be replaced by another one with a subgingival shoulder when the final prosthesis is constructed.

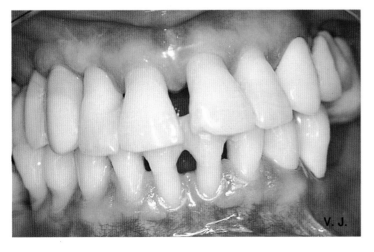

Fig. 11.17

Mouth view in maximum intercuspation. The provisionals will be used until the lower arch is treated.

XII

LABORATORY PROCEDURES FOR THE BRÅNEMARK SYSTEM

12.1 Introduction

The procedures used in the dental laboratory to construct the prosthesis will play an important role in achieving the proposed objectives. This involves the prosthodontist as coordinator and supervisor from the initial phase to the final step.

The objective will have been achieved when a balance exists between the three restorative parameters: esthetics, function, and hygiene.

The course to follow will be established jointly by the prosthodontist and the laboratory technician. Teamwork and protocol revision can only be accomplished through continuous communication by both.

Once the implants are placed, the prosthodontist and technician determine the most adequate prosthesis. This way a standard or Estheticone abutment can be chosen, or perhaps a single castable or an alumina CeraOne.

It will also be very important to follow the defined protocols. It would be damaging to alter these because of lack of communication or time.

12.2 Limiting factors

12.2.1 General aspects

The laboratory will face different cases with varying degrees of difficulty that will be defined through limiting factors.

Some of these factors will have occurred prior to laboratory processing, in other words, independent of it. Others will be a consequence of laboratory limitations. The lab technician will be responsible for correcting or minimizing these limiting factors. Sometimes the limiting factors will be irreversible, such as poor surgery, but all cases have solutions. All of the limiting factors that will be described are so important as to make the end product an overdenture instead of a fixed denture. There is no doubt that more lessons are learned from mistakes than from successes.

The limiting factors are:

• Surgery: implant placement can make it impossible to vary the treatment plan. The importance of surgery requires that it be dealt with separately.

• Patient: factors like age, sex, personality, sociocultural background, financial status, medical history, etc, can limit the treatment plan.

• Prosthodontist: He or she will detail the treatment plan from the beginning and the requirement for compliance to it. The prosthodontist's relationship with the surgeon and the lab technician will constitute somewhat of a limitation before laboratory procedures and in part during them.

• Time: A minimum amount of time will be needed for planning and treatment of each case, particularly if added difficulties arise. Frequently, the protocol is not adhered to because the time factor is not respected; in other words, the established phases are not regarded. This can occur, for example, with a VIP or a patient that lives far away, in a effort to reduce the number of appointments or advance prosthesis installment. The laboratory is responsible for allowing this to happen.

• Human and technical resources: Adequate technical resources and know-how guarantee success in most cases. State-of-the-art equipment and continuing education are a necessity. To stay abreast, it is imperative to study, attend meetings and lectures, etc, because the specialty is continuously evolving.

12.2.2 Surgery as a limiting factor

The design and construction of the prosthesis will be determined by the number and placement of implants.

The prosthodontist will have determined the treatment plan, but factors such as inexperience, isolated mistakes, or unforeseen difficulties during surgery can make modification of the preestablished treatment plan necessary.

The following factors are considered surgical limiting factors:

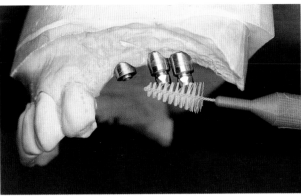

Fig. 12.1

a) Interabutment distance. To construct a prosthesis, a minimum space between abutments is needed, so as to avoid additional technical difficulties and to allow for passage of an interproximal brush for correct hygiene (Fig. 12.1). Adequate distance between implants will permit good polishing of the metal structures and will place fewer limitations on abutment selection (standard, tapered, or angulated). Apparent contours may be contraindicated with reduced posterior interabutment distance for hygienic reasons (see section 12.4.7). In partial prostheses, a variation of this factor can be an implant too close to remaining teeth or one presenting excessive convergence.

b) Abutment orientation. As an example, it can be said that a screw emerging towards the buccal of a central incisor or a canine is esthetically unacceptable (Fig. 12.2). In these cases, overdentures, angulated abutments, or even milled suprastructures will be indicated.

If the direction is somewhat unfavorable, the insertion axis can be changed through a castable chimney (see section 12.4.5). The problem is fully resolved with overdentures, but these are removable prostheses. Angulated abutments, though difficult to manipulate, are a good solution in most cases. The milled suprastructures will be used only in extreme cases due to technical complexities. The reason this grave problem occurs may lie in surgical errors or remaining bone limitations. In single implants it is rarely a problem, because the

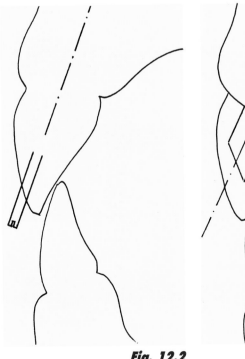

Fig. 12.2

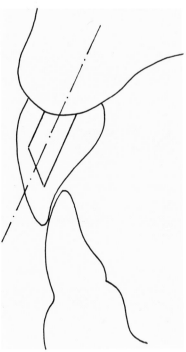

Fig. 12.3

copings (alumina, castable, or gold) are cemented (Fig. 12.3).

c) Implant position. The ideal mesiodistal position for an implant is following the axis of the tooth to be replaced. When the implant's axis shifts to the mesial or distal, an esthetic and hygiene problem is encountered; for example, with an implant placed between a lateral and a central incisor (Fig. 12.4). In the anterior segment, malpositioning is less important than inadequate abutment orientation. Here, tapered abutments are a good solution because root simulation can

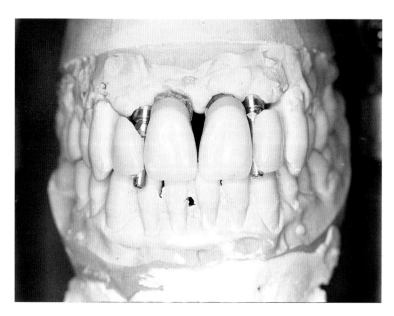

Fig. 12.4

be achieved. In the posterior segment there are fewer problems, because esthetics can be sacrificed in exchange for hygiene, as this segment is not visible while smiling.

d) Force distribution. This factor must be considered on the horizontal plane. Abutments that are too mesialized afford only a small prosthetic surface base (Figs. 12.5 and 12.6). The cantilever units would be limited to 10 mm in the maxilla and 10 to 15 mm in the mandible, thus requiring an overdenture. On the other hand, correct abutment distribution and an

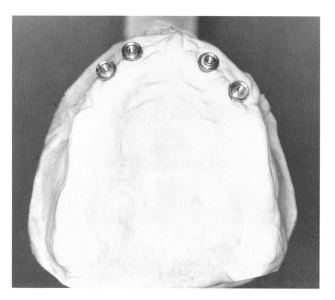

Fig. 12.5

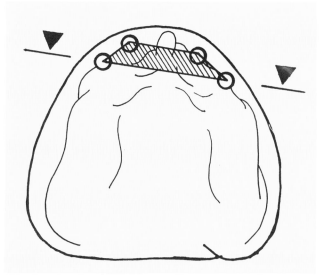

Fig. 12.6

adequate number of implants (four or five) allow for correct cantilevers that will not limit prosthesis design (Figs. 12.7 and 12.8). The smaller the cantilever, the less leverage, as determined by the two most distal abutments. To summarize, correct abutment number and distribution will permit fixed-prosthesis construction.

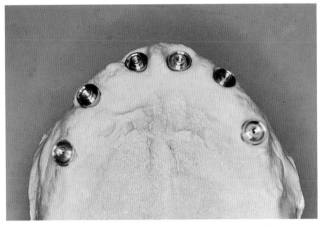

Fig. 12.7

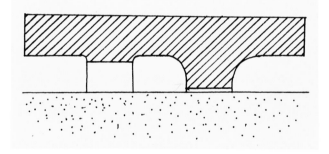

Fig. 12.8

e) Abutment height. An excessively long abutment will lead to construction and hygiene difficulties, as it requires fabrication of sharply angled instead of rounded structures (Fig. 12.9), which interfere with polishing procedures and brushing. Cemented abutments in screw-retained prostheses are an exception. Here, long abutments will ease gold-cylinder inclusion in the framework. It should not be forgotten, however, that the most anterior abutment will be overcasted (see section 12.4.8); consequently, it would be better if this abutment were short. Correcting a long abutment involves replacement by a shorter one. In partial restorations, interarch distance can be a limiting factor (Fig. 12.10).

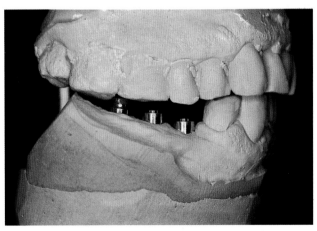

Fig. 12.9

f) Implant length. This will be most important in single implants with some kind of axial load (ie, a disoccluding canine; Fig. 12.11) or while constructing cantilevers.

Fig. 12.10

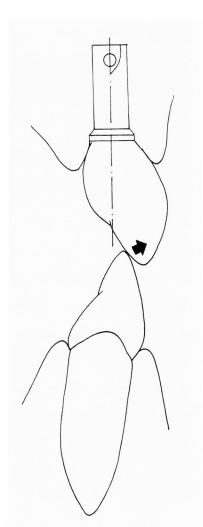

Remaining bone, its quality, and its location (maxilla or mandible) will influence this.

Two examples show how results can be improved initially by varying the abutments.

— In the first example (Figs. 12.12 and 12.13), the orientation is improved by changing from standard to angulated abutments.

— In the second example (Figs. 12.14 and 12.15), esthetics are enhanced by correcting implant positioning through substitution of a standard abutment by a tapered one.

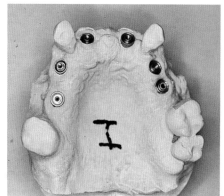
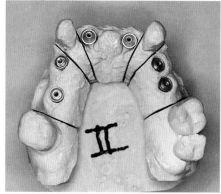

Fig. 12.11   **Fig. 12.12**   **Fig. 12.13**

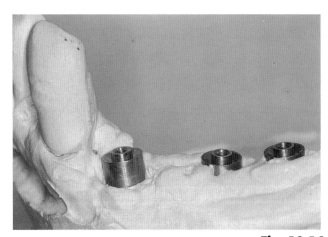
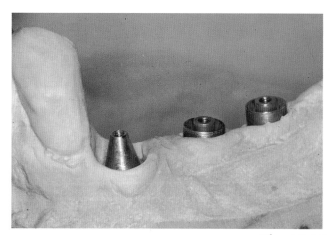

Fig. 12.14   **Fig. 12.15**

12.3 Protocols

While no two patients are the same and so no two cases are exact, it is possible to classify cases according to protocol as follows:

FIXED PROSTHESIS

3.1. Single
- Alumina
- Cast
- Overcast

3.2. Partial
- Anterior
- Posterior
- Hemiarches

3.3. Full
- Upper
- Lower
- Upper and lower

3.4. Combined
- Partial
- Full

3.5. Milled suprastructure or mesostructure
- Partial
- Full

REMOVABLE PROSTHESIS

3.6. Overdenture
- Partial
- Full

What should be done in an anterior single-tooth case or in a posterior partial prosthesis? The answer lies in defining the protocol for each type of case.

These protocols are developed in close contact with the prosthodontist and are continuously changing. This is why they must be revised frequently to conform to new materials and techniques.

Different roads can lead to the same objective, and for this reason the protocols must be somewhat flexible; the fundamentals, however, must be scrupulously followed. They are not mathematical formulas, only guidelines to be followed.

The protocols described will refer exclusively to laboratory procedures.

12.3.1 Protocol for single implants

The Brånemark system offers a single-tooth abutment, the CeraOne. This subgingival abutment, which is screw-retained to the implant, comes in five lengths (1 to 5 mm).

The laboratory must become acquainted with the three caps or copings available with the CeraOne – alumina, plastic burnout, and gold alloy for overcasting – and when each should be used.

Because of esthetics and simplicity, the alumina cap is the first choice. The only disadvantage is related to tooth size, since it does not offer good support for porcelain in large teeth (Fig. 12.16).

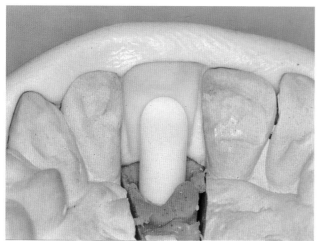

Fig. 12.16

The alumina cap can only be used with porcelain, preferably that used for jacket crowns, but care must be taken to use porcelain compatible with alumina and to avoid the use of opaquer. Since the alumina is quite clear, the cervical portion might have a low chromatic value, which can be compensated through the use of intensifiers. If opaquer should be employed, it would block out the alumina's properties, thus becoming similar to a standard porcelain-fused-to-metal crown.

Should the study waxup reveal that the alumina cap will not serve as adequate support for the porcelain, a plastic burnout cap is recommended. This type of coping is waxed up and cast following standard procedures. It has the advantage that any alloy may be used as long as it is porcelain- or acrylic-compatible.

The gold alloy coping's main advantage is its precise machining. The design allows for overcasting, and the alloy selected must have a fusion interval between 1,400° and 1,490°C to avoid deforming the cylinder during casting. The waxup and porcelain placement follow standard procedures.

The protocol for single implants is as follows:

1. The final impression shows the blue impression accessory; it can be seen because it is subgingival (Fig. 12.17). It is not necessary to have a previous impression or a customized tray.

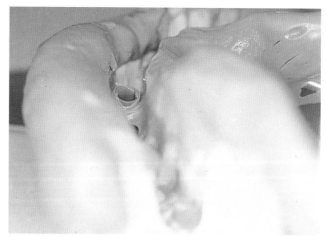

Fig. 12.17

2. After washing the impression and allowing for the working time of the material employed, the yellow plastic analog is placed into the impression accessory.

3. Before pouring the impression with hard stone, one of two steps can be followed. The first consists of lingual waxing of the junction of the two accessories (Fig. 12.18) so as to be able to verify crown fit. The second consists of pouring excess soft tissue material (Fig. 12.19), which is removed later to be tapered and shaped without undercuts, and then repositioned. Care must be taken to employ gingival material that does not adhere. Both steps may be performed simultaneously (Fig. 12.20) to have a soft tissue model with a window to check the fit.

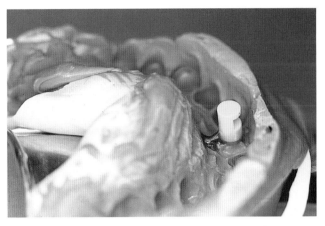

Fig. 12.18

4. Once the impression is poured with hard stone, the implant is individualized conventionally (Fig. 12.21) and the casts are then mounted on a semiadjustable articulator.

5. The appropiate coping is selected, which can be, as mentioned before:

— Alumina caps (beveled or flat).
— Burnout plastic coping.
— Gold coping for overcasting.

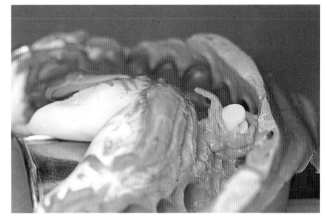

Fig. 12.19

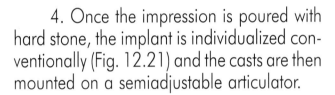

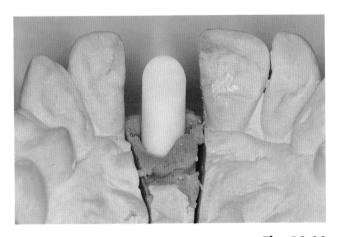

Fig. 12.20

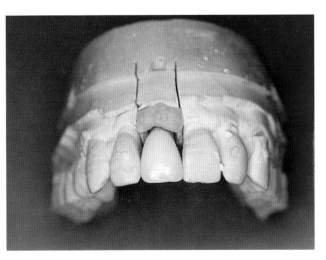

Fig. 12.21

6. If the alumina cap is selected, it must be confirmed that it serves as good support for porcelain. After that, the excess alumina is eliminated where necessary (Fig. 12.22). It should be done with a diamond disc using the index of the study waxup.

The cap then is sandblasted with non-recycled aluminium oxide and vapor cleaned. At this point, jacket porcelain can be placed, omitting the opaquer. From here on the process is the standard one using color modifiers, characterizations, preglaze try-in, makeup, and glazing.

The results are extremely attractive (Fig. 12.23, canine repositioning see chapter V, section 5.1E), even though they are more fragile than metal-supported ones. The cervical portion tends to be clear because the alumina is white. This is easily corrected with modifiers. The flat alumina caps are used in posteriors (premolars), while the beveled ones are designed for single anteriors.

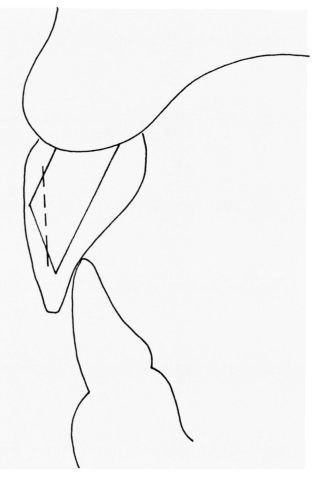

Fig. 12.22

7. Should the alumina coping prove to be insufficient for porcelain support, it is recommended to use the burnout plastic coping (Fig. 12.24). Employing the index obtained from the waxup study model, the excess plastic is eliminated (check with the opposing dentition) and wax is added until the desired contour is achieved (Fig. 12.25). The coping is cast using the preferred alloy (Ni-Cr or high gold content). This undoubtedly is an advantage. Depending on the type of material to be

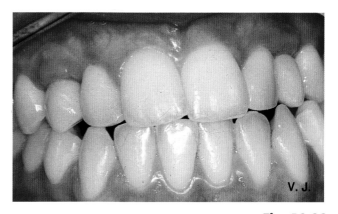

Fig. 12.23

used (porcelain or acrylic resin) the design might need modifications while building up the crown. If a guide is used on the lingual for handling or if a verification window has been created, during the preglaze try-in in the mouth the guide might compress the gingiva, so it should be removed.

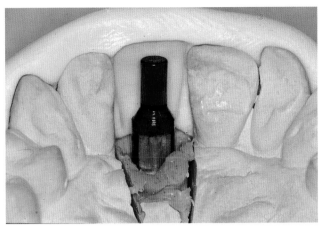
Fig. 12.24

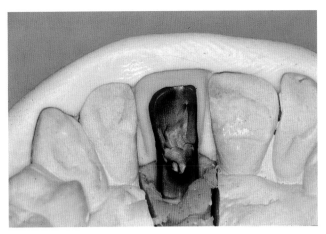
Fig. 12.25

8. The gold coping can be used for overcasting. The desired contour is developed as described in the foregoing section and is overcasted. The alloy selected should have a low fusion interval that will not damage the gold coping (1,400° to 1,490°C). The buildup follows standard procedures.

12.3.2 Protocol for partial prostheses

For the construction of implant-supported partial prostheses in anteriors, posteriors, or hemiarches, there are three types of abutments available. These are placed in the dental office. Should there be difficulties, improvements can be made by exchanging abutments. The adequate replacement should be requested.

The three types of abutments are:

— Standard
— Tapered
— Angulated

— The standard abutments come in six lengths (3, 4, 5.5, 7, 8.5, and 10 mm); they are used to build supragingival prostheses. These allow for good oral hygiene; however, esthetic difficulties may be encountered. They are recommended for posterior segments and full acrylic prostheses.

— The tapered abutments (Estheticone) are available in three lengths (1, 2, and 3 mm) and are subgingival. They are recommended for anterior segments, where esthetics are a concern, and in areas of easy access. Since they are subgingival, and if the positioning is adequate, the tooth emergence profile can be imitated. In posterior segments standard abutments are recommended.

— Angulated abutments are very versatile because they have 12 different positions. An excellent feature is that they allow a 30° change in axis insertion for the screw. The coping used for prosthesis construction is the same employed for the tapered abutment. These are recommended for abutment misalignment, and are used primarily in the anterior segment.

The protocol to be followed is:

1. The impression with the hydrocolloid copings is sent to the laboratory.

2. The impressions are poured with hard stone after fitting the respective analogs.

3. The cast is mounted on the articulator to study the case and to check abutment placement. On this model, the transfer copings are placed and splinted with acrylic resin (Figs. 12.26 and 12.27). Afterward, they are sectioned to ease tensions and are numbered for easy mouth placement. Once installed, they are splinted again with the same material. It should be considered that the three types of abutments may be used in the same impression.

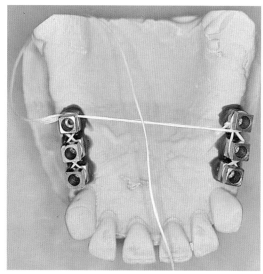 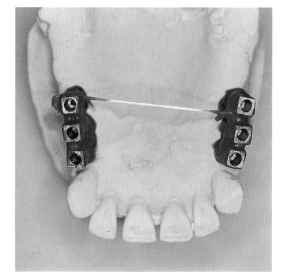

Fig. 12.26   **Fig. 12.27**

With the prepared impression accessories screw-retained to the cast, a customized tray is constructed (Fig. 12.28), creating an access window at the implant site. The tray is then delivered to the office. Some do not employ this technique, they use only hydrocolloid copings with high-density impression materials (Fig. 12.29).

4. When the final impression will be sent from the office, it is poured with hard stone after the analogs and the artificial soft gingiva have been placed (Fig. 12.30).

5. Die individualization of the master cast is done in segments, each implant-supported prosthesis must be block-sectioned. Should the implant-supported prosthesis bear attachments, it can be sectioned in two pieces (Fig. 12.31). A full implant-supported denture does not require individualization.

6. Bite registrations, especially in cantilevers, need an acrylic-resin stent. Wax boxing will

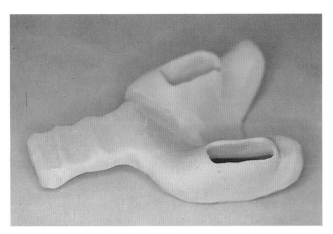

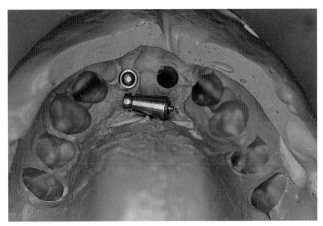

Fig. 12.28

Fig. 12.29

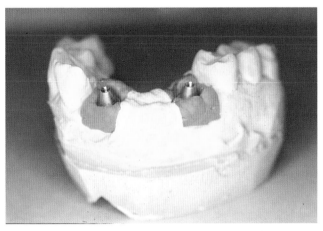

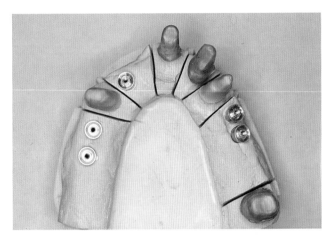

Fig. 12.30

Fig. 12.31

suffice for its construction, and acrylic resin is then poured (Fig. 12.32). Once the bite-registration stent has been constructed (Fig. 12.33) it is delivered to the office. The plate will also serve to check the validity of the master model during this first try-in. The bite-registration stent may also be fabricated by adapting light-cured materials.

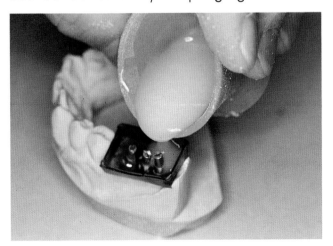

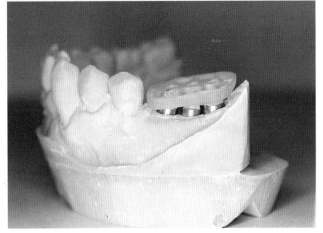

Fig. 12.32

Fig. 12.33

7. Once the master model and the opposing cast are mounted on a semiadjustable articulator, the waxup and contouring can be done in two ways:

a) Wax up the desired prosthesis (Fig. 12.34). Then cut it back until the width is adequate for porcelain placement. It is uncommon to have an acrylic-resin partial prosthesis over implants. A silicone index is of great help (Figs. 12.35 and 12.36).

b) Prefabricated teeth are mounted and joined by acrylic resin just as if we were dealing with provisionals. Then they are trimmed with discs and burs until the desired structure is

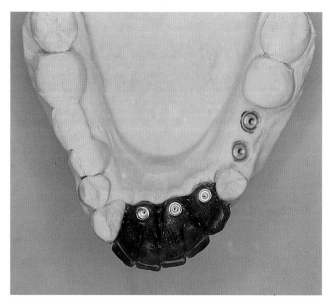

Fig. 12.34

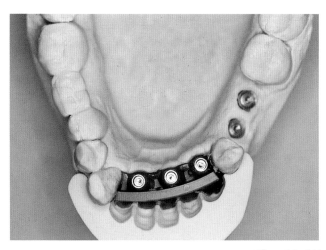

Fig. 12.35

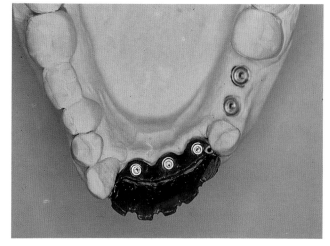

Fig. 12.36

obtained. This method is very good because it is quick and reliable in large or difficult cases (see section 12.4.6).

8. It is useful to make fine cuts between each implant after structure modeling has been completed. Once tensions disappear, it is rejoined. At this time sprues are placed (Fig. 12.37) and then it is invested. Investment expansion needs more control than in standard prostheses to obtain a passive fit.

9. Then it is cast. The abutments should be protected with wax before sandblasting to avoid surface damage (Figs. 12.38 and 12.39). If there is remaining investment on the gold cylinders, it can be cleaned easily with a fiberglass pencil. It is unacceptable to have damaged cylinders

on the abutment seating area (Fig. 12.40). The cemented-abutment technique greatly reduces this risk.

10. The sprues are cut off and the fit on the master model is checked. If it is incorrect, it can be sectioned and soldered. If the fit is good, steel protection caps are placed to refine, polish, and prepare the structure (Fig. 12.41).

It is advisable to have the clinician check the fit again. Should there be divergence, no matter how small, it is sectioned again, splinted with Duralay, and then soldered.

The solder repair is a valid one, and in fact sometimes frameworks are constructed in segments to be soldered later on. All these difficulties are solved with the cemented-abutment technique.

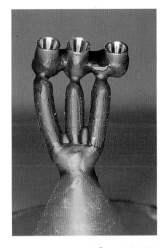

Fig. 12.37

11. The framework is then covered with porcelain following standard procedures. The protective caps must always be used when refining porcelain and polishing either with discs or burs to avoid damaging the seats of the abutments. On occasion, the cylinders contact porcelain and become stained green. The causative agent is silver, which is not equally present in all porcelain brands. Certain products are available to avoid this (nongreening liquids). The standard cylinders have 24.5% Ag, while the tapered have 14.5% Ag.

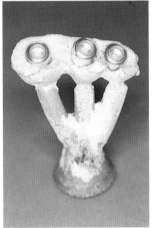

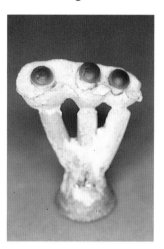

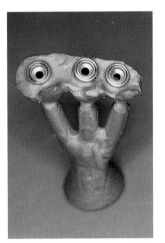

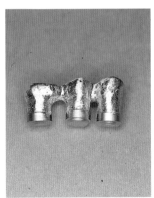

Fig. 12.41

Fig. 12.38   **Fig. 12.39**   **Fig. 12.40**

12.3.3 Protocol for full prostheses

Full prostheses will be either upper or lower, though both may occur in the same case. This would be a full-mouth restoration, which requires special attention to the occlusion.

The specific profiles of the edentulous maxilla and mandible demand certain implant orientation (Figs. 12.42 and 12.43). For this reason, porcelain is used on the upper and acrylic resin on the lower. Depending on which is used, the design will vary drastically.

A) Protocols for full fixed porcelain prostheses

1. The first impression is poured, then studied, and prepared with the final impression accessories. A customized tray is also built.

2. The final impression will be poured in hard stone, but the soft tissue model is constructed before this, especially when dealing with subgingival tapered abutments. The dies will not be trimmed (individualized) whatsoever. However, this may be done in those areas where precision attachments will be used.

The bite-registration stent is constructed over the standard or tapered cylinders. This may be done through wax boxing or by adapting an acrylic-resin light-cured base (Fig. 12.44). It is then delivered to the office for intraoral registrations.

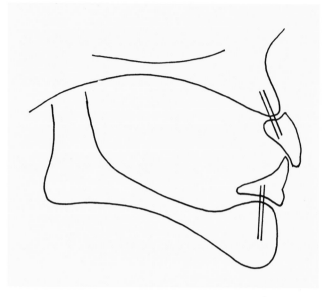

Fig. 12.42

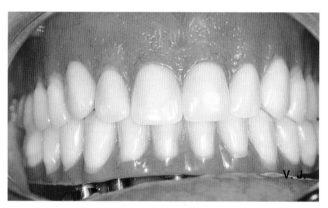

Fig. 12.43

3. The prosthodontist registers the occlusal record and takes a face bow and other wax registrations to mount the case on a semiadjustable articulator. All other pertinent information, such as the midline, vertical dimension, smile line, color, etc, is recorded. At this stage, the relationship between the prosthodontist, patient, and technician becomes very important. A duplicate of the patient's full denture (Fig. 12.45) will offer information about the shape, size, and positioning of teeth, as well as about vertical dimension and occlusion, if all of these are to be maintained.

4. The case is now mounted on the articulator with all the necessary data and with a set of teeth selected in accordance with the denture duplicate. Acrylic-resin tooth mounting is begun, similar to full-denture mounting (Fig. 12.46). In this fixed prosthesis, anterior or canine guidance is built in; this is also done when dealing with a fixed opponent or an implant-supported overdenture. Should the opponent be a conventional full denture that is not going to be substituted, a balanced occlusion is indicated.

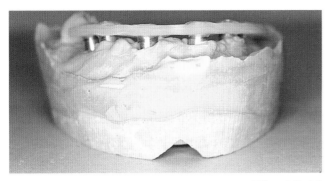

Fig. 12.44

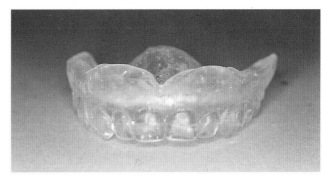

Fig. 12.45

Once the teeth have been arranged, a silicone index is taken and relined with acrylic resin, thus becoming similar to a provisional (Fig. 12.48). This must be contoured and polished with the protection caps on. It is then ready for office try-in, which will be done this time by the technician in person. This is necessary to gain more information from the try-in.

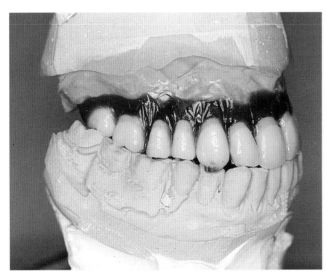

Fig. 12.46

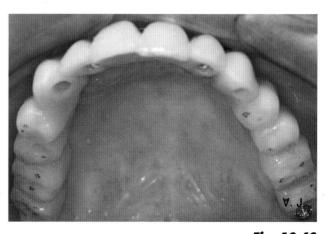

Fig. 12.47

5. The prosthodontist tries in the acrylic-resin model and adjusts the occlusion. New registrations are taken. The midline and smile line are checked and the patient's approval is obtained (Fig. 12.48). If necessary, further corrections are made until it is satisfactory. The technician then returns to the laboratory to start the framework.

6. In the laboratory, the new centric relation registrations must be the first thing checked.

Fig. 12.48

A customized anterior guide table is constructed in self-curing acrylic resin, registering the lateral and protrusive movements on the articulator (Fig. 12.49). These have previously been adjusted in the mouth. Consequently, a customized guide is developed and a silicone index is obtained of the tooth waxup. The waxup will be cut back with discs and burs (Fig. 12.50) to obtain the framework. This technique is simple and reliable. The attachments are placed with the help of a surveyor, and the angles are then rounded off with wax.

It is recommended to section between each implant to control tensions (Fig. 12.51). The opponent is checked against the index to verify the presence of enough space for porcelain placement.

7. The wax framework will now require the placement of sprues, investment material and casting.

8. Once cast, the framework is sandblasted following the precautions described previously and then checked for fit on the master cast (Fig. 12.52). This verification requires the removal of the artificial soft gingiva, especially in tapered abutments.

9. A try-in is advised at this time. If the adjustment is not adequate, the prosthodon-

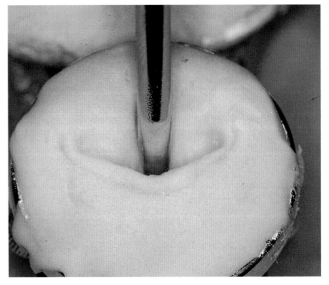

Fig. 12.49

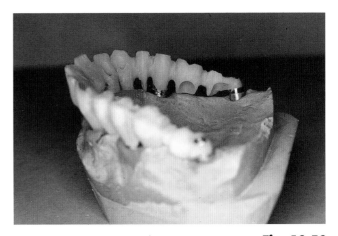

Fig. 12.50

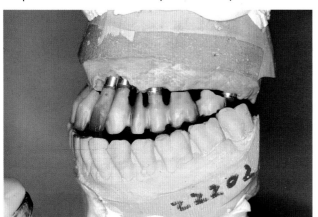

Fig. 12.51

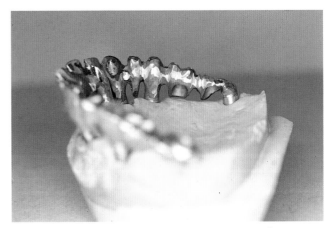

Fig. 12.52

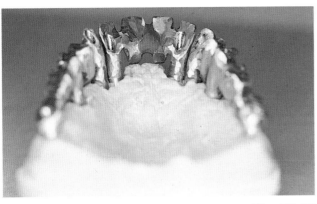

Fig. 12.53

tist will section it and join the segments with acrylic resin to be soldered in the laboratory (Fig. 12.53). Soldering is a valid repair and is not a problem in itself.

10. Refining, polishing, and structure preparation is always done with the protection caps on and tightly screwed to the cylinders. Once the structure is fixed to the master cast (Fig. 12.54), the silicone index is used again for a final check on the space available for porcelain placement.

11. The porcelain placement with opaquer and porcelain plus the characterizations follows standard procedure. However, it must be considered that cervical esthetics will sometimes be compromised because of gingival retraction, which will make teeth look longer (Fig. 12.55). This can easily be corrected with removable artificial gingiva (Fig. 12.56). It should also not be forgotten that green stains may appear in the cervical region, which can be controlled with nongreening liquid. The protection caps must always be placed on the cylinders when polishing porcelain.

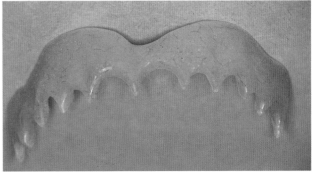

Fig. 12.54

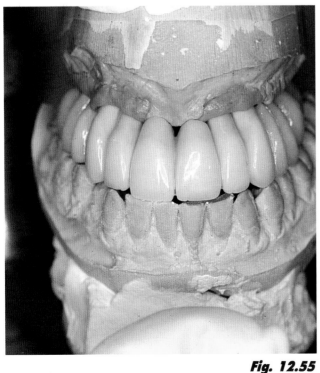

Fig. 12.55

Fig. 12.56

The makeup, glazing, and polishing are not any more difficult than in standard porcelain procedures.

B) Protocol for full fixed acrylic-resin prostheses

1. The initial impression, customized tray, and transfer for the final impression have been described previously.

2. The final impression is poured in hard stone after placing the standard analogs. This kind of prosthesis requires standard abutments. Once the master cast is obtained, the gold cylinders are placed and an acrylic-resin stent for bite registration is constructed and delivered to the office.

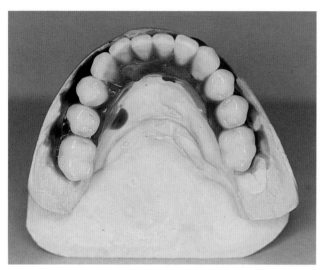

Fig. 12.57

3. The dental office will return to the laboratory the registrations, vertical dimension, midline, smile line, and face bow for mounting on a semiadjustable articulator. Any other necessary information will also be sent.

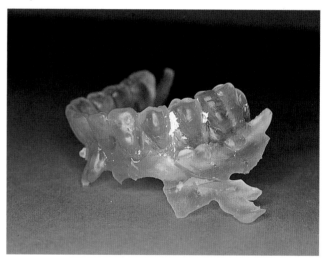

Fig. 12.58

4. With the aid of the full-denture duplicate, the teeth are selected according to size and shape. The teeth are mounted similarly to full-denture teeth (Fig. 12.57). If the opponent is fixed, the occlusal scheme will include canine or anterior guidance. Should the opponent be a full denture, a balanced occlusion would be indicated.

5. The mounted teeth are duplicated with clear acrylic resin (Fig. 12.58) to be trimmed to the desired framework shape. This technique will make contouring easier.

6. The necessary copings are prepared with burnout acrylic resin (Fig. 12.59) for

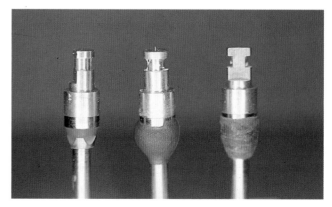

Fig. 12.59

casting with the cemented-abutment technique. This is not the only procedure, but it is the best for achieving a passive fit through an easy and simple technique. Since the copings are not commercially available, they must be fully constructed in the laboratory (see section 12.4.8).

7. The copings are transfered to the master cast and all checked with the acrylic-resin duplicate that previously has been trimmed and fixed to the opponent (Fig. 12.60).

8. A sheet of wax is shaped into a horseshoe form with access holes over the implants (Fig. 12.61). It will serve as support during the framework waxup.

9. The wax base will serve to join the copings, using the same material employed to construct them (Figs. 12.62 and 12.63). Once it is stable (free of tension), it can be handled easily and safely.

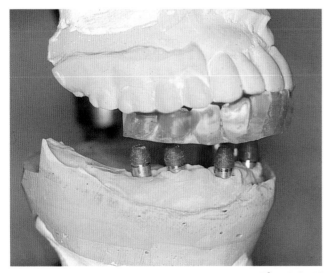

Fig. 12.60

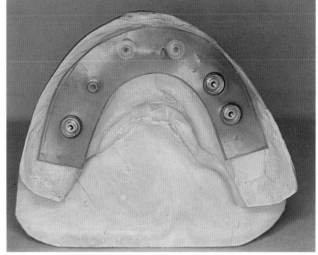

Fig. 12.61

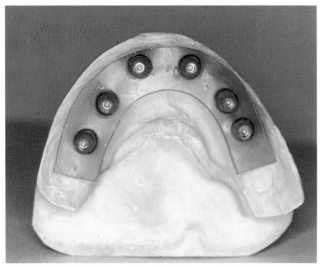

Fig. 12.62

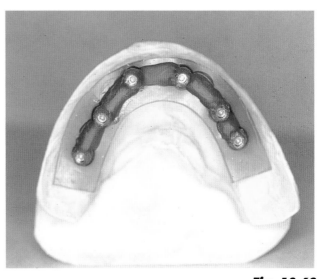

Fig. 12.63

10. Framework design is begun, building up the periphery following the clear acrylic-resin index (Fig. 12.64). The cantilevers should touch the gingiva, leaving space for distal implant hygiene. The profiles should be convex or, in some cases, flat.

11. Once the contouring is finished and before placing the retentions, the correspondence is checked with the acrylic-resin index. This will help decide where to place the retentions (Fig. 12.65).

12. When the acrylic-resin retentions have been developed, it is now ready for sprue placement and investing (Figs. 12.66 and 12.67).

The most mesial gold cylinder is left incorporated into the framework for overcasting. Its function is to serve as a reference during installment and to resist maximum traction.

13. Following casting, it is sandblasted, taking care not to damage the gold cylinder, which can be protected simply by covering it with wax (Fig. 12.68).

14. The sprues are cut off, and the framework is refined and polished (Fig. 12.69). This single cylinder must be protected by the steel cap. Cylinder fit is checked on the master cast.

15. The polishing paste is cleaned off first with detergent and later with water vapor. It is then silanized or tin-plated where the acrylic resin will be placed (Fig. 12.70).

16. Pink-colored opaquer is applied to avoid metal translucency (Fig. 12.71).

17. Pink wax is used when mounting the teeth. Now it is ready for the final try-in (Figs. 12.72 and 12.73).

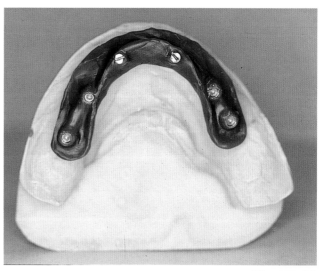

Fig. 12.64

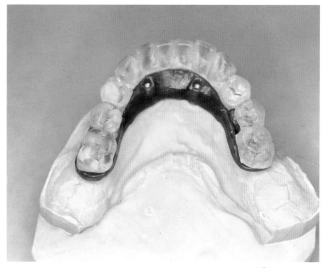

Fig. 12.65

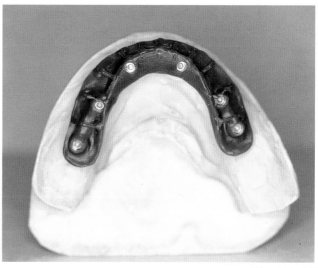

Fig. 12.66

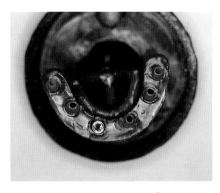

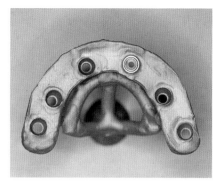

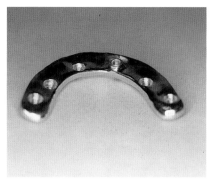

Fig. 12.67   Fig. 12.68   Fig. 12.69

18. If no corrections are needed, it is placed in the flask and processed following standard procedures. When it is polished and completed, it is delivered to the office for abutment cementation. Anaerobic composite resin is used for this.

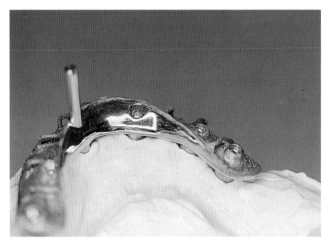

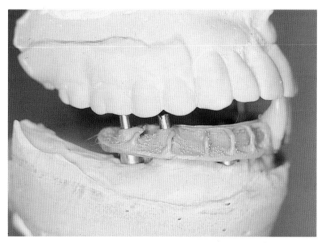

Fig. 12.70   Fig. 12.71

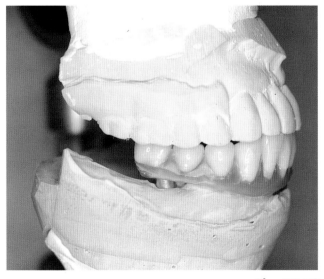

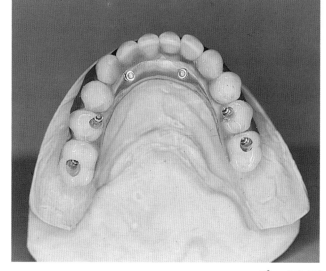

Fig. 12.72   Fig. 12.73

In cases of full oral restoration (upper and lower), the prefabricated teeth would be mounted according to standard full-denture procedures. However, canine or anterior guidance is recommended. Balanced occlusion is not indicated because they are fixed prostheses. Using one arch as a reference, the opponent is then constructed. It is important to obtain patient lateral and protrusive registrations (Figs. 12.74, 12.75, 12.76, and 12.77).

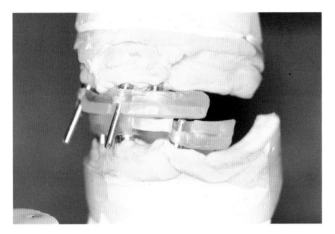

Fig. 12.74

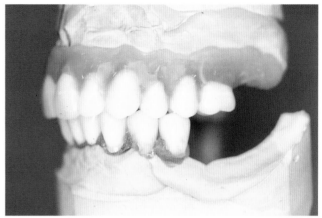

Fig. 12.75

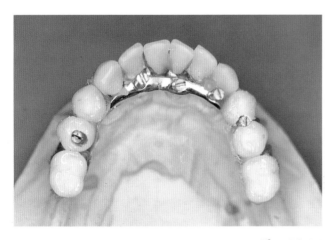

Fig. 12.76

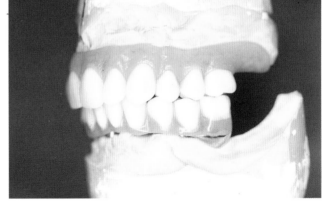

Fig. 12.77

12.3.4 Protocol for combinations

Combinations are implant-supported prostheses that also use remaining natural dentition for support (Figs. 12.78 and 12.79).

While designing the prosthesis, it should be remembered that implants are rigid and the teeth have resilience. The prosthesis is constructed with attachments, customized milling, screws, stress-relievers, or telescopic crowns.

Depending on the implants, these prostheses can be partial or full. A total combined prosthesis over implants is one that lacks stress-relievers or similar attachments, though it may use milling or telescopic crowns (Figs. 12.80 and 12.81).

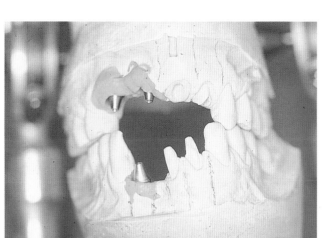

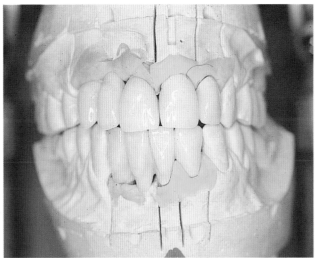

Fig. 12.78

Fig. 12.79

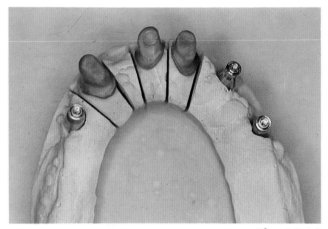

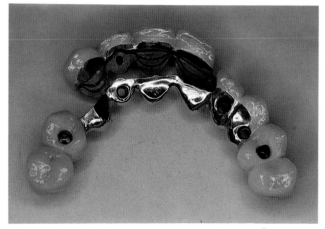

Fig. 12.80

Fig. 12.81

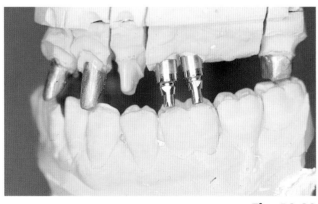

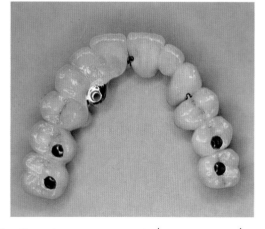

Fig. 12.82

Fig. 12.83

Totals and partials require die individualization to reconstruct the prepared remaining teeth (Fig. 12.82 and 12.83). Care must be taken to leave each implant group as a block to avoid errors.

An example of this kind of treatment is the construction of a provisional removable prosthesis with attachments, while osseointegration is taking place.

The attachments will serve later to relate the implant prosthesis to the remaining teeth (Figs. 12.84, 12.85, and 12.86).

The protocol is similar to that of partials, in combination with standard techniques such as the surveyor, customized milling, attachments, etc.

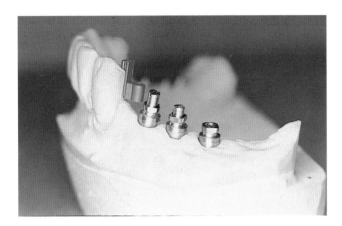

Fig. 12.84

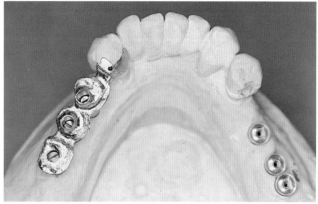

Fig. 12.85

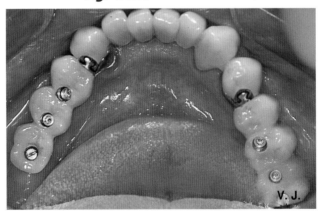

Fig. 12.86

12.3.5 Protocol for milled suprastructures

A milled suprastructure consists of an infrastructure and suprastructure that fit perfectly and can be joined by screws or springs. Artificial gingiva is not necessary because the structure can be removed for hygiene purposes, and the prosthesis would then be an overdenture with a more or less sophisticated bar.

This structure is usually used to correct lack of abutment parallelism that cannot be solved through angulated abutments (Fig. 12.87).

Protocol

The first steps (impression-taking, pouring, preparation, cast articulation) are the same as those described previously.

1. The infrastructure is waxed up and anatomically contoured, regardless of implant orientation (Fig. 12.88).

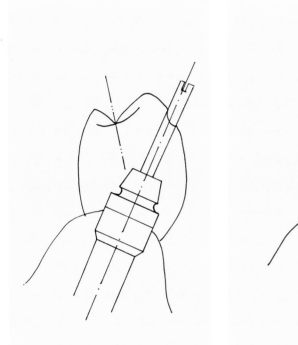

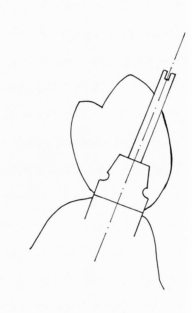

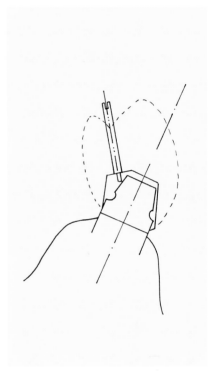

Fig. 12.87   **Fig. 12.88**   **Fig. 12.89**

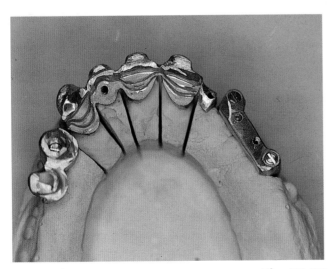

Fig. 12.90

2. The infrastructure is made parallel, cut back, and milled. The attachments or springs are placed in favorable areas, taking care to leave room for the suprastructure and porcelain or acrylic resin (Fig. 12.89).

3. The infrastructure is then cast, refined, and polished (Fig. 12.90). Protective steel caps should always be used.

4. A full waxup is done again and later is cut back to the desired suprastructure. An acrylic-resin burnout shaft is of great help. Observe closely the suprastructure's screw and sheath (Figs. 12.91 and 12.92).

5. Standard porcelain placement is followed. Before polishing, the protective caps are placed and the contours of the screw-retained suprastructure and infrastructure are evened. Finally, they are polished (Fig. 12.93).

12.3.6 Protocol for overdentures

The external design for overdentures is similar to that of conventional full dentures. The difference lies in the anchoring

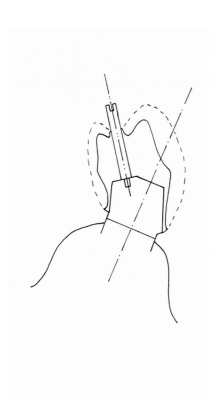

Fig. 12.91

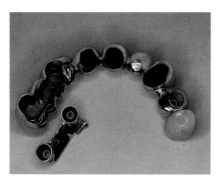

Fig. 12.92

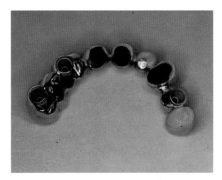

Fig. 12.93

mechanism, which thanks to implants is very solid. The anchoring is achieved through bars or ball-type mechanisms, which allow for a smaller prosthesis palate, in turn resulting in added patient comfort.

Protocol

1. The standard analogs are screwed to the final impression (Fig. 12.94). Standard abutments are used because they are supragingival and thus are easier to handle. Tapered abutments are not necessary, because the overdenture will cover them. The previous steps have already been described. Once the final impression is poured, it is important to have a detailed cast, which sometimes will require boxing. The impression is poured a second time; this cast will be used for soldering the clips and attachments to the suprastructure, which will be described further on.

2. At this stage, the type of bar to be used is determined. It can be cast, cast and milled, or soldered (Fig. 12.95).

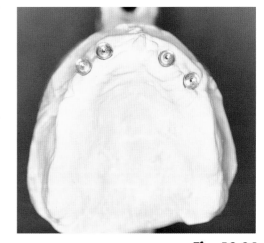

Fig. 12.94

The course of action selected will partly depend on the prosthodontist, the number of implants, and the technician's preference. Undoubtedly, soldered bars permit better adjustment. The castable bars use burnout material and are cast to the gold cylinders and attachments selected. The bars used are Dolder, Ackerman, cylindrical, etc, with their pertinent clips. The cast bars may be milled for guidance or retention. The soldering bars are prefabricated. As a general rule, the gold cylinders are splinted to the bars. The clips are

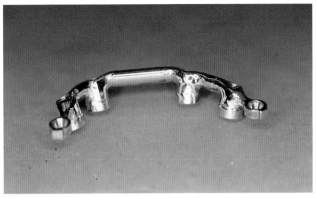

Fig. 12.95

placed on the anterior segment that lacks resilience, so they act as reciprocals. The attachments are placed in the distal part of the posterior cylinders. A fulcrum will be determined by the attachments; consequently, resilient attachments and clips are recommended. Rigid attachments increase the risk of fracture and poor function (Figs. 12.96 and 12.97).

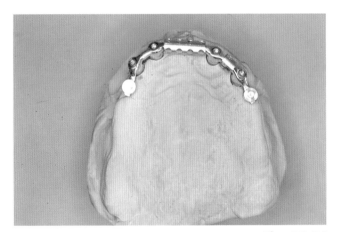

Fig. 12.96

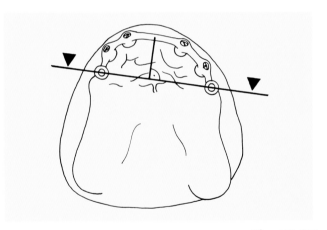

Fig. 12.97

3. Constructing castable bars follows standard procedures for core casting. The only precaution to be aware of is alloy selection. The alloy should not damage the gold cylinders or attachments, so a fusion interval of 1,280° to 1,350°C is recommended.

However, more care must be taken in soldered bars. The final result is very good, with excellent passive fit, and good mechanical behavior.

The solder should have a fusion interval of 100° to 200°C lower than the cylinders, bars, and attachments to avoid damaging them. The heat treatment, which is done last, must also be considered.

Here is an example (Figs. 12.98 and 12.99)

ACCESSORIES	FUSION INTERVAL	TREATMENT	COLOR
Cylinder DCA 072	1,280° – 1,350°C	Self-hardened	White
Dolder Bar C + M	880° – 940°C	15 min at 400°C	Yellow
Ceka attachment Pallax	980° – 1040°C	15 min at 500°C	White
Ceka Sol Solder	810° – 840°C	—	Yellow

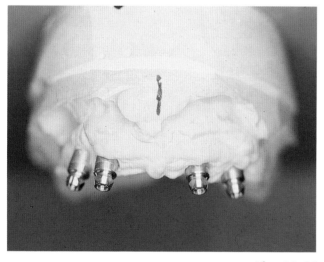

Fig. 12.98

Fig. 12.99

4. The bars and attachments are placed with the help of a surveyor and are glued with burnout acrylic resin (Figs. 12.100 and 12.101). The bar is reinforced in the middle (Fig. 12.102) by, for example, an old bur, which is joined by burnout acrylic resin. It must all be firmly fixed by screws, leaving enough time for tensions to stabilize (Fig. 12.103)

5. Bar preparation for soldering requires its removal from the master cast, substituting

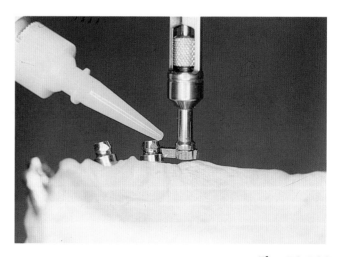

Fig. 12.100

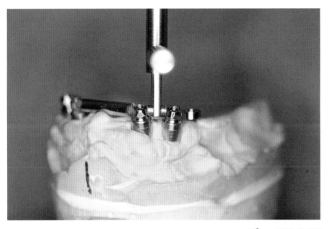

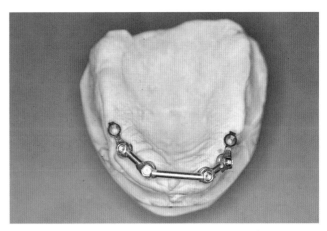

Fig. 12.101   Fig. 12.102

gold screws for steel ones, then firmly screwing in the analogs. The steel screw used is a laboratory working screw.

With the abutments in place, the bar is then embedded in plaster (Fig. 12.104).

6. Once the stone plaster has set, the complex is unscrewed and the auxiliary bar is removed. Wax is added to those areas where investing should be avoided and the bar is again screwed into the plaster. It is all covered with 63% phosphate investment, leaving openings for soldering (Fig. 12.105). This technique produces excellent results. The investment delays plaster degradation while plaster controls investment expansion.

7. It is introduced into the cylinder oven at 300°C for 30 minutes to allow gases to exit and to reach an adequate temperature for soldering with a torch.

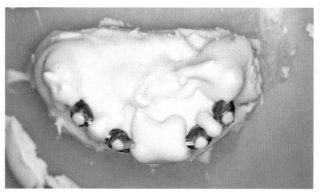

Fig. 12.104

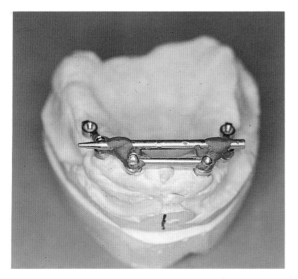

Fig. 12.103   Fig. 12.105

8. A soft and fine oxypropane flame is used to solder the elements to each other. This will be done quickly and deliberately, avoiding flame damage.

9. When cool (Fig. 12.107), the investment is removed carefully, cleaning the attachments and cylinders with a fiberglass pencil. It should not be sandblasted, and its fit on the master cast must be checked. If the fit is incorrect, it is sectioned where necessary and the process is repeated (Fig. 12.108). If the color of the cylinders is uniform and shiny, the soldering process is correct. Blackened cylinders or cylinders with stains indicate that excessive heating has occurred.

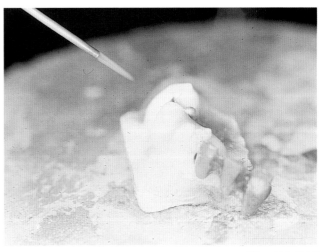

Fig. 12.106

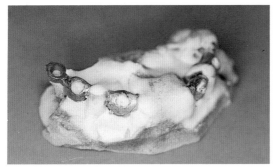

Fig. 12.107

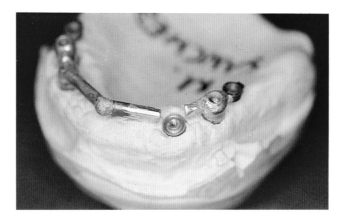

Fig. 12.108

The protective caps are placed and excess solder is removed. Magnifiers can help avoid damage to the margins. Slightly polish with rubber wheels and pumice; the protective caps must be kept on (Fig. 12.109). When the prosthesis is completed, it is polished, remembering that polishing is a wear-producing procedure. It is now checked in the mouth.

10. If. the try-in has been satisfactory, the overdenture's suprastructure is designed. The bar is retained by screws to the master cast, and the nonresilient clips and the resilient patrixes are placed where they belong (Fig. 12.110). Plastic attachments and clips have to be replaced frequently. They perform poorly compared to metal ones.

11. A sheet of wax is used to cover everything, similar to the removable-partial-denture

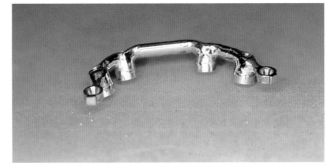

Fig. 12.109

technique, leaving the saddle stops, the clips, and attachments wax-free, to be soldered. Bar parallelism should be observed (Fig. 12.111).

12. The cast is duplicated, with the wax serving as a spacer, and it is poured with investment.

13. The prepared investment cast is ready for suprastructure waxup. First the bar is covered, leaving an opening in the places to be soldered (Fig. 12.112). The rest is designed with the aid of prefabricated elements (Fig. 12.113). When dealing with full maxillary cases, palatal coverage is not indicated. There is no real need for this, and the patient will be more comfortable. This process is similar to partial removable denture (PRD) construction.

14. The sprues are placed; then it is invested and cast. The alloy must have adequate mechanical properties. PRD common alloys and palladium-based ones are adequate selections.

15. Once it is sandblasted, the sprues are cut off, leaving the rest untouched except for the parts to be soldered (Fig. 12.114). This

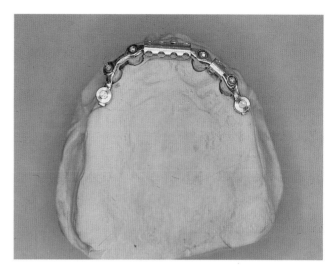

Fig. 12.110

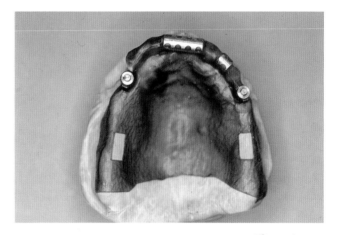

Fig. 12.111

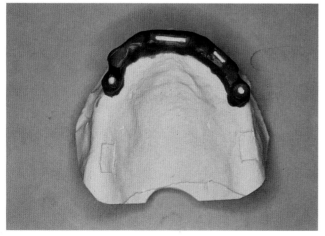

Fig. 12.112

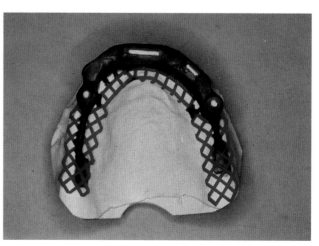

Fig. 12.113

is only done here because light polishing helps solder flow, while roughened surfaces decrease flow.

The suprastructure is placed on the master cast to check its fit (Fig. 12.115).

16. The suprastructure is now soldered to the clips and attachments. This is all done

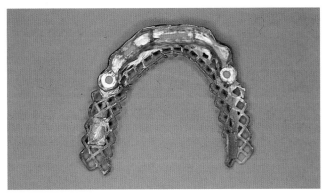

Fig. 12.114

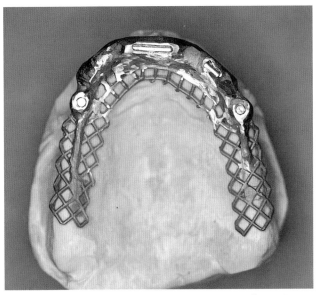

Fig. 12.115

on the second cast obtained from the final impression. This plaster cast will control suprastructure expansion, but afterward it will be ineffective for further use (Figs. 12.116 and 12.117). The bar has already been tried in. When soldering, the bar is retained to the cast by steel screws so as to avoid damaging the gold ones.

17. Once milled, the acrylic stops are placed on the saddles for bite registration. It is delivered to the office, where bite registrations, midline, smile line, tooth color, and tooth shape are recorded. The lab technician should be present during the try-in. The full-denture duplicate will provide permanent information.

18. The acrylic resin used for the bite registration is removed and the framework is cleaned, first with detergent and then with

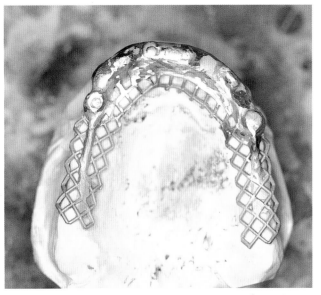

Fig. 12.116

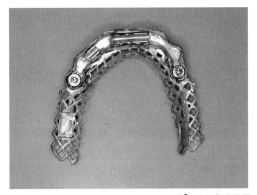

Fig. 12.117

vapor. The next step is to tin-plate or silanize for pink-opaquer application (Fig. 12.118).

19. Once the casts are mounted on the semiadjustable articulator, tooth placement with pink wax is begun (Fig. 12.119). Canine or anterior guidance is developed, unless the opponent is a conventional full denture. Bal-

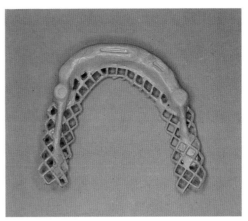

Fig. 12.118

anced occlusion is indicated in that case.

20. The waxup is tried in. If the patient is satisfied, the prosthesis can be completed. The denture is flasked following standard procedures.

The bar will be polished once more; however, each polishing causes wear, and this may interfere with both clip and attachment precision.

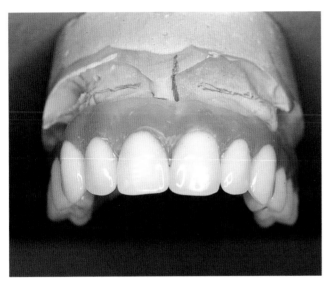

Fig. 12.119

12.4 Laboratory procedures

12.4.1. Soft tissue model impression pouring

Conventional prostheses over prepared teeth first require pouring the impression; the die is then individualized and prepared, and construction of a soft tissue model from a silicone index (Fig. 12.120) is then performed.

However, in implant-supported prostheses, the process is reversed. The analogs are positioned firmly (singles) or screwed (standard and tapered) (Fig. 12.121) in the impres-

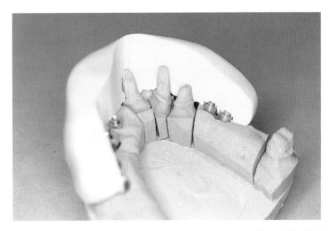

Fig. 12.120

sion; later the masking gingiva is poured around the analogs. It is then removed in a block and the gingiva is trimmed to a tapered shape to avoid plaster mechanical retention (Fig. 12.122). Some gingival materials (eg, elastomers) are trimmed easily with a hot blade.

The tapered gingival block is placed again in the impression (Fig. 12.123) and hard stone plaster is poured following standard procedures (Fig. 12.124). The gingival material used should not adhere to the stone but should be held in place firmly.

An old technique, that is still valid, is placing wax around the analog-transfer joint. Afterward, a buccolingual bridge is waxed up. This will create a window on the cast that will permit cylinder fit examination.

This procedure can be combined with the soft tissue model technique (fig. 12.125).

These techniques must be used in cases that employ subgingival abutments. Other abutments only need to add wax around the

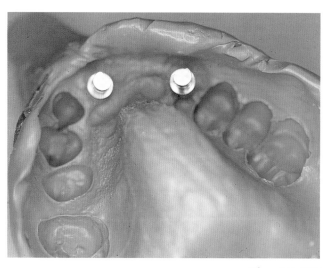

Fig. 12.121

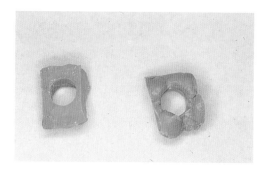

Fig. 12.122

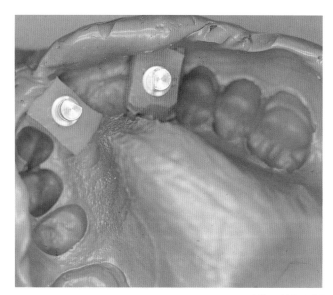

Fig. 12.123

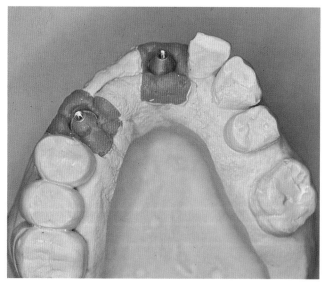

Fig. 12.124

analog and impression coping interface, followed by pouring.

12.4.2 Full-denture duplication

By using a duplicating device (Fig. 12.126) and alginate, an impression of the patient's denture is obtained. Acrylic resin is poured and the duplicate (Fig. 12.127) thus produced is very useful is conveying information such as vertical dimension, midline, shape and size of teeth, etc. It is of great help to the technician at all times (Fig. 12.128).

12.4.3 Bite registrations (stents)

These can be partial or total, but the construction procedure is the same. There are two methods for building bite stents.

One system is by wax-boxing the abutments (Fig. 12.129); the box formed is then

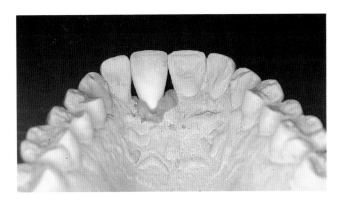

Fig. 12.125

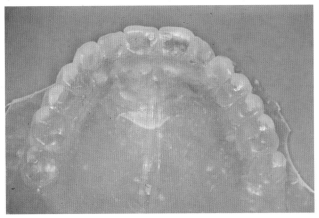

Fig. 12.127

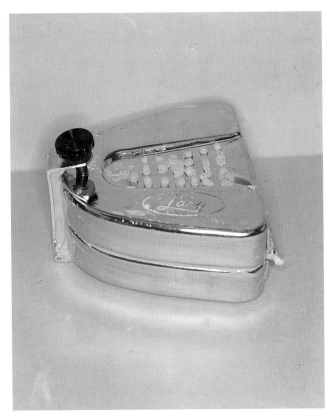

Fig. 12.126

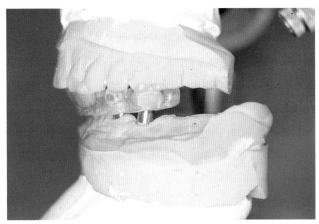

Fig. 12.128

poured with clear acrylic resin (Fig. 12.130). It is left in place for 30 minutes to allow for tensions to stabilize, and afterward is contoured. Positioning grooves or retentions are prepared, and it is placed back on the master cast and delivered to the office for registration procedures (Fig. 12.131). It will also serve as the first test for cast precision; this is why clear acrylic resin is recommended.

The other method consists of adapting light-cured acrylic resin (Fig. 12.132) to the cylinders, which is then photopolymerized

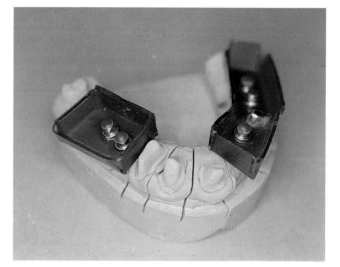

Fig. 12.129

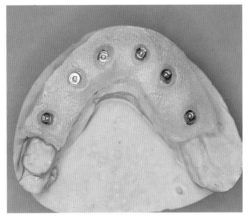

Fig. 12.130

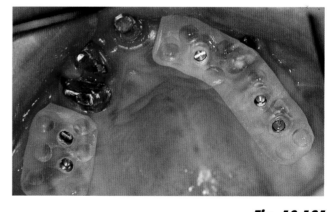

Fig. 12.131

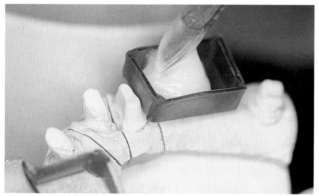

Fig. 12.132

(Fig. 12.133). Afterward, it is trimmed and occlusal retention for the registration material is carved (Fig. 12.134). The rest of the protocol is the same.

12.4.4 Acrylic-resin burnout sheath

In full fixed prostheses, the sheath is used to reinforce the gold cylinders or the burnout

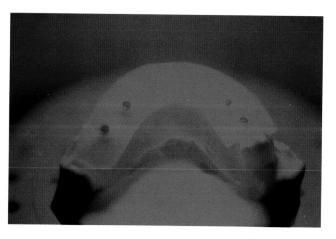

Fig. 12.133

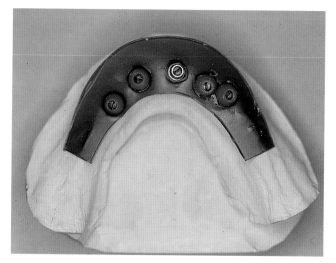

Fig. 12.134

Fig. 12.135

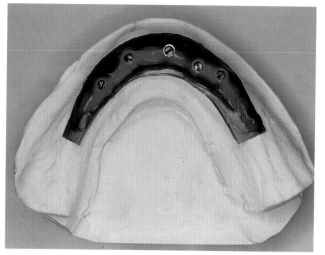

Fig. 12.136

type (cemented abutments) (Figs. 12.135 and 12.136) on the waxed-up framework. This makes handling the master cast easier and safer.

During partial prosthesis waxup, it has a similar function, but it also positions the plastic chimneys (Fig. 12.137).

In milled suprastructures, telescopic prostheses, and customized milling it serves as support for the suprastructure and allows for

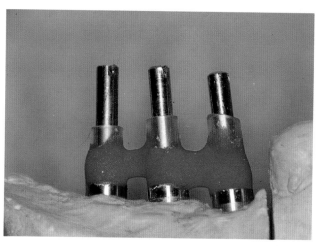

Fig. 12.137

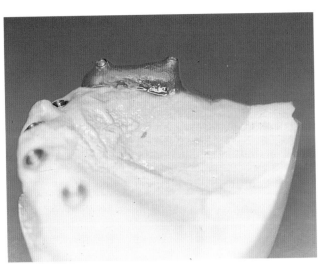

Fig. 12.138

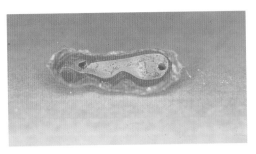

Fig. 12.139

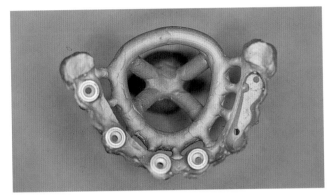

Fig. 12.140

predictable reproduction of angles or delicate forms (Figs. 12.138, 12.139, 12.140). The acrylic resin must burn out completely without leaving residues and its contraction should be controllable.

12.4.5 Castable chimneys

These are castable plastic sheaths with an inner diameter slightly larger than the steel working screws. The purpose of the plastic sheath is to simplify chimney construction during framework waxing procedures (Fig. 12.141). In theory, it also serves as guidance for slight changes in the insertion axis.

This change in insertion must be moderate (Figs. 12.142 and 12.143) to allow screwdriver access. If the change in axis has to vary significantly, angulated abutments or milled suprastructures would be needed.

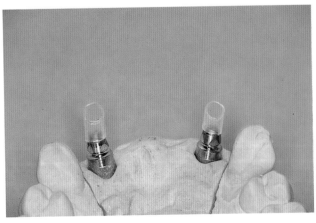

Fig. 12.141

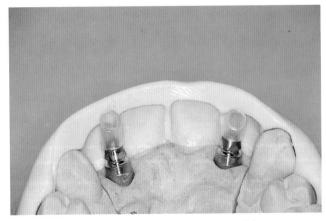

Fig. 12.142

12.4.6 Framework construction from modeled acrylic resin

First, a study model is constructed with prefabricated acrylic teeth (Fig. 12.144). Once the teeth are mounted and a silicone index is taken (Fig. 12.145), this is relined with acrylic resin similarly to provisionals (Fig. 12.146).

A buccal index is also obtained for use as a reference while contouring the framework.

In the patient, the occlusion, midline, smile line, etc are corrected (see 10.3).

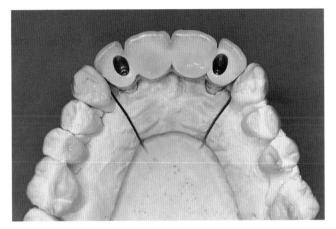

Fig. 12.143

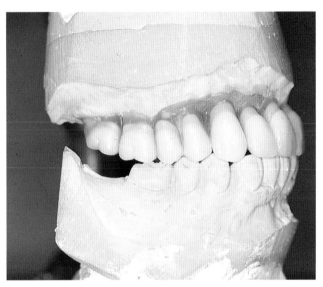

Fig. 12.144

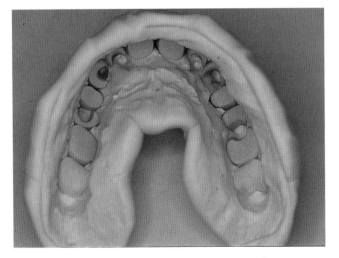

Fig. 12.145

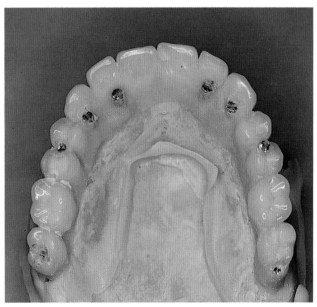

Fig. 12.146

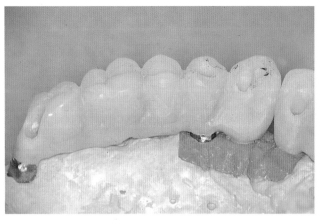

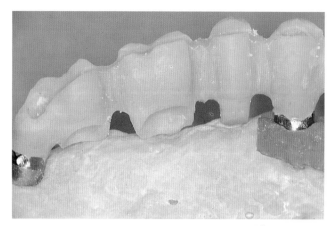

Fig. 12.147 *Fig. 12.148*

After all the corrections have been done, the acrylic resin is cut back until a framework with enough space for porcelain placement is obtained (Figs. 12.147 and 12.148). This procedure is done with discs and burs. The buccal silicone index is very useful to check the space available for the porcelain. To break acrylic-resin tensions, it must be sectioned between implants.

Wax is added to round off angles and a final check with the opponent is carried out. The acrylic-resin framework is now ready for spruing and casting (Figs. 12.149 and 12.150).

12.4.7 Apparent contours

In implant-supported prostheses, the tooth-emergence profile should start at the gingiva without compromising mesiodistal anatomy, making hygiene easy. A well-positioned implant and a tapered abutment will make this simple to do. However, if the implant is too lingualized, this will be difficult following standard procedures.

An optical illusion will solve this problem. In a mesiodistal view, the anatomical contours can be seen, maintaining enough buccolingual space for adequate hygiene (see chapter VI, section 6.6.2).

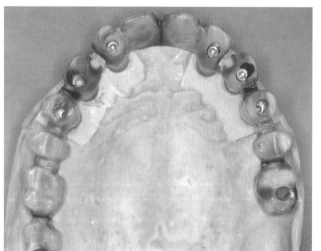

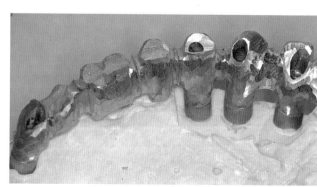

Fig. 12.149 *Fig. 12.150*

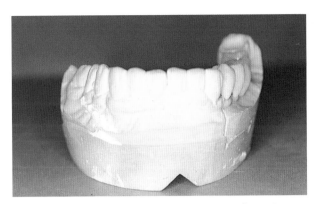

Fig. 12.151

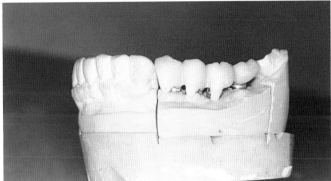

Fig. 12.152

This can be achieved by constructing a droplike extension which will serve as the anatomical contour when viewed mesiodistally, thus hiding the large embrasures (dark spaces between teeth; Fig. 12.151). While constructing it, the access for hygiene is checked with an interproximal brush. This is only an esthetic solution, so the number of drop or tear extensions to be placed will depend on how far back they can be seen when the patient smiles widely. This makes hygiene of the distal areas easier (Fig. 12.152).

12.4.8 Cemented abutments

This is an excellent technique to achieve a passive fit. It consists of constructing copings that will be cemented in the mouth, obtaining a full passive fit.

Copings for this technique are not commercially available yet, so they must be fully constructed in the laboratory.

The construction begins by placing the gold cylinder on the analog and retaining it by a longer screw. The cylinder's undercuts are blocked with wax. Then it is covered by castable acrylic resin and once it has set, it is contoured at low speed (Fig. 12.153). The rest of the procedure for prosthesis construction has already been described (see section 12.3.3).

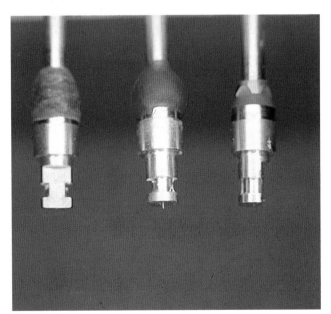

Fig. 12.153

When the prosthesis is completed and the patient has approved it, the areas to be cemented are tin-plated. Excess anaerobic acrylic cement is removed easily, but care must be taken not to scratch the framework with sharp instruments. The most difficult thing to achieve in casting procedures is a passive fit. This problem is easily resolved and is simple to carry out in the laboratory.

12.4.9 Sprue placement and investing

There are two different case-types: large structures (full) or small structures (partial). The large structures consist of one piece per arch (Fig. 12.154), while small ones or segmented structures will not be supported by more than three or four implants (Fig. 12.155), thus making passive fit easier to achieve.

These problems do not exist in cemented frameworks (Fig. 12.156).

Not more than three sprues will be necessary for casting implant framework because its width serves as a diffusion bar. The sprues can be short and thick (4 mm). If more than three sprues are used, a bar should be placed to avoid deformities. The thickness of the framework can cause backflow porosity, especially at the cast-cylinder interface.

If circular diffusors are used in full-prosthesis casting, the distal area should be sectioned

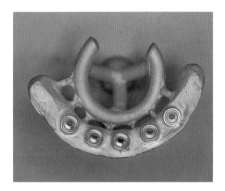
Fig. 12.154

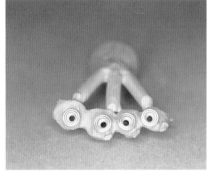
Fig. 12.155

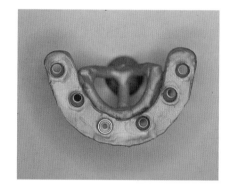
Fig. 12.156

to avoid distortions at the ends of the framework during casting (Fig. 12.157). This is a predictable technique, particularly if the centrifugal casting machine is not strong.

The framework should be placed in the ring away from the thermic center and it should follow its curvature. Consequently, the sprues are placed lingually. Paper and elliptical casting rings should not be employed.

Investment concentration will also be extremely important. Standard investment for

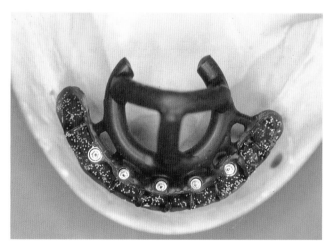
Fig. 12.157

porcelain- or acrylic-compatible alloys is used. Personal knowledge and experience can be useful for handling the different investment materials available, as well as during investing procedures and sprue placement.

Special care must be taken to control investment expansion. This depends on so many factors that it is impossible to make specific recommendations.

These factors are:

— Room temperature.
— Hygroscopic setting.
— Investment brand.
— Water-liquid ratio.
— Adequate storage.
— Laboratory machinery and its condition.
— Speed of temperature rise, and oven stop intervals for preheating.
— Metal or plastic rings and casting ring liners.

Experience shows us that the phosphate-bonded investments should have a concentration of 63% when using plastic casting rings.

To conclude, there are two laws that should be considered:

— The error margin is directly proportional to the distance between abutments. In other words, the longer the distance between abutments, the greater the lineal expansion error.
— The error margin is directly proportional to the number of abutments. In other words, the more abutments placed, the greater the possibility of torsional error.

12.4.10 Standardization of screws

The use of screws to hold the prosthesis (see sections 12.3.4 and 12.3.5) has been discussed elsewhere. However, while testing or checking the prosthesis, two or three different types of screws may be used. When recalling the patient, it can be even more difficult, plus the armamentarium and screwdrivers will have to be expanded.

This can be avoided by standardizing the screws, using the same type on the suprastructure as the ones employed for holding the infrastructure to the implants.

This can be done by having the necessary accessories:

— A 1.2-mm cylindrical bur for the handpiece.
— A manual 1.4-mm male diestock.

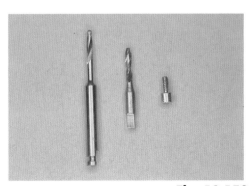

Fig. 12.158

Nothing else will be needed for threadmaking. Before casting, the infrastructure must be perforated with the 1.2-mm bur (Fig. 12.159) in the designated area for screw placement. Careful investing is advised to obtain the drilled hole in the cast. Once cast, the infrastructure is drilled with the 1.2-mm bur on low speed to eliminate porosities and residual investment (Fig. 12.160).

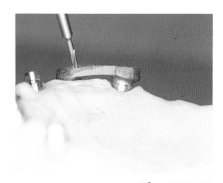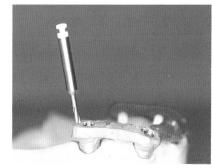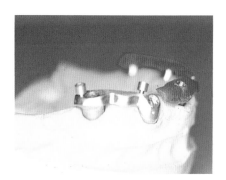

Fig. 12.159   *Fig. 12.160*   *Fig. 12.161*

The thread is made manually with the 1.4-mm male diestock (Fig. 12.161). Now the suprastructure can be waxed up according to screw placement.

12.4.11 Soldering processes

Passive fit is especially sensitive to soldering techniques, because soldering joins two framework segments, whether sectioned on purpose or during a repair.

The main problem is controlling linear expansion in implant-supported prostheses. The linear expansion is unavoidable when heating an alloy (with torch or oven), so the use of some kind of means to limit the expansion is required.

The following three types of soldering procedures for implant-supported prostheses will be detailed:

1. Soldering of porcelain framework (torch).
2. Post soldering for porcelain-fused-to-metal prostheses (oven).
3. Low-fusion soldering of acrylic-resin structures and bars.

1. Investment preparation at 63% concentration follows standard routine. However, the investment will have a longitudinal frame made of steel bars (for example, old burs) included to control expansion and other distortions.

If a plaster base is used to control the expansion, new steel analogs (standard and tapered) must be used, because ordinary analogs will melt during soldering. Both methods can be used jointly.

The soldering is performed with a fine-tipped torch. If high-fusion soldering is used, the technique is a "pseudosoldering" one. If the solder used is from the same alloy to be soldered, it constitutes an autogenous solder. This second type is much more difficult to do.

2. The preparation for this type of soldering is similar to standard oven procedures. Expansion is controlled through steel bars and steel analogs, as described previously.

3. Since this method is low fusion, soldering plaster may be used to control expansion. The conventional analogs may also be used. The complete soldering procedure can be found in section 12.3.6.

12.5 Alloys

The selection of an alloy for implant-supported prostheses depends primarily on the use of acrylic resin or porcelain. The preferred alloy is used, but it must meet two requirements:

1. The fusion interval must be low enough to not damage the implant cylinders when overcasting.

2. The alloy must not be sensitive to backflow porosity during cooling, as these frameworks are always quite thick. The thickness avoids resistance problems.

The cylinders and caps (copings) used for the Brånemark system are:

— Alumina caps.
— Burnout single copings.
— Gold single cylinders.
— Gold cylinders.
— Gold cones.

Porcelain is placed directly on the alumina cap. This technique follows standard procedures, so it will not be described.

Burnout singles offer the advantage that gold alloys or Ni-Cr–based alloys may be used.

The three other types of cylinders will now be described, beginning with the fusion interval and their composition so as to be able to compare them to different commercial alloys.

CYLINDERS	FUSION INTERVAL	COMPOSITION
Standard DCA 072, DCA 073	1280°–1350°C	39.5% Pt, 26% Pd, 24.5% Ag, 10% Au
EsthetiCone DCB 141	1400°–1490°C	60% Au, 20% Pd, 19% Pt, 1% Ag
CeraOne DCA 160, DCB 160	1400°–1490°C	60% Au, 20% Pd, 19% Pt, 1% Ag

The comparisons between implant cylinders and commercial alloys require the knowledge of the fusion interval and composition of four known alloys.

CATEGORY AND INDICATION	FUSION INTERVAL (°C)				
	BRAND 1	BRAND 2	BRAND 3	BRAND 4	SUMMARY
	(C & M)	(METALOR)	(JELENKO)	(ELEPHANT)	
Alloys for Porcelain					
I High Au Content 75%	1050–1140 1125–1240	1070–1165 1125–1240	1020–1130 1150–1260	1050–1150 1145–1255	1020–1260
II High Precious Metal Content 75% Au + Gr Pt	1160–1320 1240–1305	1180–1300 1120–1235	1345	1145–1225 1240–1300	1145–1300
III Pd Based 50% Pd	1130–1230 1190–1270	1145–1270 1160–1280	1190–1270	1115–1240 1190–1230	1115–1280
Alloys for Acrylic Resin					
IV High Au Content > 68% Au	910–960 1075–1110	910–965 960–1060	895–925	890–945 900–975	895–1110
V High Precious Metal Content 50% Au + Gr Pt	815–895 1055–1090	865–890 870–925	860–910 960–1030	860–900 950–1070	815–1090
VI Ag Based Pd, Au: > 38% Ag 25% > Au + Gr Pt	860–910 1160–1200	875–1035 990–1045	910–960	940–965 1020–1100	860–1200
Basic Alloy					
VII Ni–Cr Based	—	1250–1290	1125–1275	—	1225–1290

NOTE: The fusion interval (melting interval) of each brand represents first the lowest melting point of the alloy and second the highest melting point of the alloy.
- The summary of fusion intervals contains the lowest and highest melting points of the four brands.
- Platinum metal group (Gr Pt): Au, Pt, Pd.

The following are the conclusions reached when comparing the cylinder and alloy tables:

1. With respect to the fusion interval:

— All of the cylinders are compatible with categories I (porcelain) and IV, V, and VI (acrylic resin).
— The alloys II, III, and VII must be studied individually to avoid damaging the cylinders, with a 100°C safety margin.

2. With regards to the composition:

— None of the cylinders belongs to high Au content (I and IV) nor Pd (III and VI) nor basic alloys (VII).
— All gold cylinders belong to categories II and V, but their values are closer to categories III and VI.
— The Ni-Cr alloys should be discarded because they do not match the precious metal with regards to backflow porosity.

To summarize, gold cylinders of the CeraOne and EsthetiCone systems can be used with any alloys from category I to VI. The Ni-Cr should not be used because of the tremendous difference with the cylinders. The Ni-Cr alloys are used with burnout copings.

The gold cylinders are compatible with palladium-based alloys (III and VI) and high precious-metal content alloys (II and V). If porcelain is to be used, a nonsilver alloy, categories II and III, is recommended.

If acrylic resin is to be employed, categories V and VI (palladium-silver–based) are advised.

The author's choice is:

— For porcelain: palladium-based alloys free of silver (III).
— For acrylic resin: palladium-silver–based alloys (VI).

It should not be forgotten that the abutments are made of pure titanium. This metal has excellent biocompatibility, and will control ionic interchange between different metals because it is a poor conductor of electricity. The following form measures show this.

PHYSICAL AND MECHAN- ICAL PROPERTIES	UNITS	TITANIUM	BERYLLIUM	IRON
Melting Point	°C	1,660	1,278	1,535
Thermal Conductivity (between 20°–100°C)	W/mK	17	175	71
Electrical Relative Conductivity	% respect Cu	4	42.5	17.5
Electrical Resistance	$\mu \Omega$ cm	42	4	9.7

BIBLIOGRAPHY

OCCLUSION

Arnold NR. Tratamiento oclusal. Buenos Aires: Inter-Médica, 1978.

Barghi N, Dos Santos J, Narendran S. Effects of posterior teeth replacement on temporomandibular joint sounds: a preliminary report. J Prosthet Dent 1992;68:132-136.

Benito Vicente MC. Valor de la imagen por Resonancia Magnética en las alteraciones dinámicas de la ATM [Master's thesis]. Madrid: UCM Faculty of Dentistry, 1992.

Bossman AE. Hinge axis determination of the mandible [Thesis]. Utrecht, The Netherlands: University of Utrecht, 1974.

Campos Ortega A. Centro de Estudios Estomatológicos de la III Región. Spain: Reunión en Murcia, 1987.

Casado Llompart JR. Personal communication, 1992.

Curnutte D. Personal communication, 1980.

Curnutte D. Course on occlusion. College of Dentistry of Madrid, 1981.

Davies PL. Electromyographic study of events for forward head posture. J Craniomand Pract 1979;1:49-59.

DeBoever J. Functional disturbances of the temporomandibular joint. In: Zarb GA, Carlsson GE (eds). Temporomandibular Joint: Function and Dysfunction. Copenhagen: Munksgaard, 1979:193-201.

Farrar WB. Differentiation of temporomandibular joint dysfunction to simplify treatment. J Prosthet Dent 1972;28:629-636.

Friedman MH. Anatomic relations of the medial aspect of the temporomandibular joint. J Prosthet Dent 1988;59:495-498.

García Villaescusa A. Personal communication, 1993.

Gross MD. La Oclusión en Odontología Restauradora: Técnica y Teoría. Buenos Aires: Labor, 1982.

Hamerling J. Mandibular movement patterns, a methodological and clinical investigation of children with lateral forced bite [Thesis]. Amsterdam: University of Amsterdam, 1983.

Hansson T, Oberg T, Carlsson GE, Kopp S. Thickness of the soft tissue layers and the articular disk in the temporomandibular joint. Acta Odontol Scand 1977;35:37.

Hansson T. Temporomandibular changes related to dental occlusion. In: Solberg WK, Clark GT (eds). Temporomandibular Joint Problems. Biologic Diagnosis and Treatment. Chicago: Quintessence, 1980:129.

Hansson T, Honee W, Hesse J, Jiménez V. Disfunción Craneomandibular. Barcelona: Praxis, 1988.

Helkimo M, Ingervall B, Carlsson GE. Variation of retruded and muscular position of the mandible under different recording conditions. Acta Odontol Scand 1971;29:423.

Huffman R, Regenoüs J. Principles of Occlusion. London, Ohio: H&R Press, 1973.

Kaplan AS, Assael LA. Temporomandibular Disorders: Diagnosis and Treatment. Philadelphia: Saunders, 1992.

Katz, GT. The determinants of human occlusion. Los Angeles: Marina Press, 1972.

Kobayashi Y, Hayasgu K, Stohler CS. Experimental occlusal interference and amount of the Bennett movement [abstract 25]. J Dent Res 1982;61:47.

Korbendam A, Abjean J. Oclusión (Aspectos Clínicos, Indicaciones Terapéuticas). Buenos Aires: Panamericana, 1980.

Krough-Poulsen W. The significance of occlusion in temporomandibular function and dysfunction. In: Solberg WK, Clark GT (eds). Temporomandibular Joint Problems. Biologic Diagnosis and Treatment. Chicago: Quintessence, 1980:93.

Lauritzen AG: Atlas de Análisis Oclusal. Madrid: Martínez de Murguía HF Editores, 1977.

Linek Dos HA. Tooth carving manual. Los Angeles: University of Southern California School of Dentistry.

López Alvarez JL. Personal communication, 1991.

Lundberg M, Welander U. The articular cavity in the temporomandibular joint: A comparison between the oblique lateral and tomographic image. Medica-Mundi 1970;15:27.

Magnusson T, Enbom L. Signs and symptoms of mandibular dysfunction after addition of balancing side interference. Acta Odontol Scand 1984;42:129-135.

Martínez Ross E. Personal communication, 1980.

Martínez Ross E. Oclusión Orgánica. Barcelona: Salvat, 1985.

Martínez Ross E. Rehabilitación Temporomandibular. Aparato Ortopédico Intermaxilar. Mexico: Cuéllar, 1992.

McCall CM, Szmyd L, Ritter RM. Personality characteristics in patients with temporomandibular joint symptoms. J Am Dent Assoc 1962:66:694.

Michael CG, Javid NS, Colaizzi FA, Gibbs CH. Biting strength and chewing forces in complete denture wearers. J Prosthet Dent 1990;63:549-553.

Miralles R, Bull R, Manns A, Roman E. Influence of balanced occlusion and canine guidance on electromyographic activity of elevator muscles in complete denture wearers. J Prosthet Dent 1989;61:494-498.

Mongini F. The importance of radiography in the diagnosis of TMJ dysfunctions. A comparative evaluation of transcranial radiographs and serial tomography. J Prosthet Dent 1981;45:186.

Morgan D, Hall W, Vamvas J: Enfermedades del Aparato Temporomandibular. Buenos Aires: Mundi, 1979.

Noder Merhy H. Oclusión orgánica y su influencia en la odontología [Thesis]. Mexico, 1977.

Okeson JP. Long-term treatment of disk-interference disorders of the temporomandibular joint with anterior repositioning occlusal splints. J Prosthet Dent 1988;60:611-616.

Okeson JP. Management of TM Disorders and Occlusion. St. Louis: Mosby, 1989.

Randow K, Carlsson K, Eddlun J, Oberg T. The effect of an occlusal interference on the masticatory system. An experimental investigation. Odontol Rev 1976;27:245-253.

Sarnat BG, Laskin DM. The Temporomandibular Joint. A Biological Basis for Clinical Practice, ed 3. Springfield, IL: Charles C Thomas Publisher, 1980.

Solberg W, Nordstrom B, Bibb C, Forsythe A, Hansson T. Malocclusion associated with TMJ changes in young adults at autopsy. J Dent Res 1985;64(special issue):151-164.

Solnit A. Personal communication, 1980.

Solnit A, Curnutte DC. Occlusal Correction: Principles and Practice. Chicago: Quintessence, 1988.

Stuart C. Personal communication, 1980.

Travell JG, Simons DG. Myofascial Pain and Dysfunction. The Trigger Point Manual. Baltimore, MD: Williams and Wilkins, 1984.

Weinberg LA. Temporomandibular joint function and its effect on centric relation. J Prosthet Dent 1973;30:176-195.

IMPLANTS

Albrektsson T, Bergman B, Folmer T, et al. A multicenter study of osseointegrated oral implants. J Prosthet Dent 1988;60:75-84.

Albrektsson T, Lekholm U. Osseointegrated dental implants. Dent Clin North Am 1986;30:165-172.

Badanelli Rubio L. Consideraciones oclusales in prótesis fija sobre implantes osteointegrados [Thesis]. Madrid: UCM Faculty of Dentistry, 1991.

Baker JL, Goodking R. Precision Attachment Removable Partial Dentures. St. Louis: Mosby, 1981.

Balshi T. Resolving esthetic complications with osseointegration using a double casting prosthesis. Quintessence Int 1986;17:281-287.

Brånemark P-I, Zarb GA, Albrektsson T. Tissue-Integrated Prostheses: Osseointegration in Clinical Dentistry. Chicago: Quintessence, 1985.

Brewer AA, Morrow RM. Overdentures. St. Louis: Mosby, 1980.

Brygider R. Precision attachment-retained gingival veneers for fixed implant prostheses. J Prosthet Dent 1991;65:118-122.

Cibirka RM, Razzoog ME, Lang BR, Stohler CS. Determining the force absorption quotient for restorative material used in implant occlusal surfaces. J Prosthet Dent 1992;67:361-364.

Clinical Research Associates Newsletter. 1990;4(March):3.

Cox JF, Zarb GA. Alternative prosthodontic superstructure design. Swed Dent J 1985;28(suppl):71-75.

Díaz-Arnold AM, Jons RA, LaVelle WE. Prosthodontic rehabilitation of the partially edentulous trauma patient by using osseointegrated implants. J Prosthet Dent 1988;60:354-357.

El Charkawi H, El Wakand B, Naser ME. Modification of osseointegrated implants for distal extension prostheses. J Prosthet Dent 1990;64:469-472.

Ericsson I, Lekholm U, Brånemark P-I, Lindhe J, Glantz P-O, Nyman S. A clinical study evaluation of fixed bridge restoration supported by the combination of teeth and osseointegrated titanium implants. J Clin Periodontol 1986;13:307-312.

Gasca Muñoz F. Personal communication regarding Panavia, 1990.

Gates WD, Diaz-Arnold AM, Aquilino SA, Ryther JS. Adhesive strength to tin plated and non-tin plated alloys [abstract 1379]. J Dent Res 1992;71 (special issue):278.

Goll GE. Production of accurately fitting full-arch implant frameworks: Part I-Clinical procedures. J Prosthet Dent 1991; 66:377-384.

Haas M, Wegscheider WA, Bratschko RO, Permann R, Kudera F. Le proceda silicoanter ameliore-t-il a laison resine-metal? Quintessence Zahntech 1986;11:1191-1199.

Henry PJ. An alternative method for the production for accurate casts and occlusal record in osseointegrated implant rehabilitation. J Prosthet Dent 1987;58:694-697.

Imbery TA, Davis RD, et al. Evaluation of tin plating systems for a high-noble alloy. Int J Prosthodont 1993;16:55-59.

Jiménez V, Torroba P. Diseño de prótesis sobre implantes para conseguir un ajuste pasivo: Técnica del cilindro cementado sobre prótesis atornilladas. Actualidad Implantológica 1992;1(5):27-32.

Jones SD, Jones FR. Tissue-integrated implants for the partially edentulous patient. J Prosthet Dent 1988;60:349-357.

Jörnéus L. Avoiding overload in single-tooth restorations. Nobelpharma News 1992;6(4):3.

Jörnéus L, Jemt T, Carlsson L. Loads and designs of screw joints for single crowns supported by osseointegrated implants. Int J Oral Maxillofac Implants 1992;7:353-359.

Kunenberg IJ, Murray GM. Design of superstructures for osseointegrated fixtures. Swed Dent J 1985;28(suppl):63-69.

Langer B, Sullivan D. Osseointegration: Its impact on the relationship of periodontics and restorative dentistry, Part 1. Int J Periodont Rest Dent 1989;9:85-107.

Leung N, Zarb GA, Pilliar R. Castings of prosthetic superstructures in tissue integrated dental prostheses. J Dent Res 1983;62:292-301.

Leung N, Zarb GA, Watsson P. Non gold alloy system for prosthetic frameworks. J Dent Res 1982;62:324-329.

Lewis S, Sharma A, Nishimura R. Treatment of edentulous maxillae with osseointegrated implants. J Prosthet Dent 1992;68:503-508.

Linkow LJ, Rinaldi AW, Weiss WW, Smith GH. Factors influencing long-term implant success. J Prosthet Dent 1990;63:64-73.

Loos LG. A fixed prosthodontic technique for mandibular osseointegrated titanium implants. J Prosthet Dent 1986;55:232-242.

López Alvarez JL. Técnicas de Laboratorio en Prótesis Fija. Madrid: Goya, 1987.

Lundquist S, Carlsson GE. Maxillary fixed prostheses on osseointegrated dental implants. J Prosthet Dent 1983;50:262-271.

Lytle J, Skurow H. An interdisciplinary classification of restorative dentistry. Int J Periodont Rest Dent 1987;7(3):8-41.

Martínez Corriá R. Personal communication, 1991.

Martínez Ross E. Procedimientos clínicos y de laboratorio de Oclusión Orgánica. Bogota, Colombia: Ediciones Monserrate, 1984.

McCarney JW. Cantilever rest: An alternative to the unsupported distal cantilever of osseointegrated implant-supported prostheses for the edentulous mandible. J Prosthet Dent 1992;68:817-819.

McKinney R, Steflik D, Koth D. Evidence for a functional epithelial attachment to ceramic dental implants. J Periodontol 1985;56:579-591.

Naert I, Quirynen M, van Steenberghe D, Darius P. A six-year prosthodontic study of 509 consecutively inserted implants for the treatment of partial edentulism. J Prosthet Dent 1992;67:236-245.

Olins P, Hill Elaina M. Tensile strength of air abraded tin plated metal luted with three cements [abstract 974]. J Dent Res 1991;70(special issue):387.

Omula I, Yamouchi J, Harada I, Wada T. Adhesive and mechanical properties of a new dental adhesive [abstract 561]. J Dent Res 1984;63(special issue):233.

Parel SM. Modified casting technique for osseointegrated fixed prosthesis fabrication: A preliminary report. Int J Oral Maxillofac Implants 1989;4:33-40.

Parel SM. The SmiLine System. Dallas, TX: Taylor Publishing, 1991.

Preiskel HW. Ataches de precisión en odontología. Buenos Aires: Mundi, 1977.

Preiskel HW. Precision Attachment in Prosthodontics: The Applications of Intracoronal and Extracoronal attachments (vols 1 and 2). Chicago: Quintessence, 1984.

Quirynen M, Naert I, van Steenberghe D, Nys L. A study of 589 implants supporting complete fixed prostheses. Part 1: Periodontal aspects. J Prosthet Dent 1992;68:655-663.

Rasmussen EJ. Alternative prosthodontic techniques for tissue integrated prostheses. J Prosthet Dent 1987;57:198-204.

Richter E-J. Basic biomechanics of dental implants in prosthetic dentistry. J Prosthet Dent 1989;61:602-609.

Rieger MR, Mayberry M, Brose MO. Finite element analysis of six endosseous implants. J Prosthet Dent 1990;63:671-676.

Rossen IP, Braak LH, de Putter C, de Groot K. Stress-absorbing elements in dental implants. J Prosthet Dent 1990;64:198-205.

Salagaray VL. Implantes inmediatos transalveolares. Madrid: Biomedical Function, 1992.

Santamaría Zuazua J, Gill Lozano J, Magdaleno Quintanal F, Estefanía Cuncín E, Barbier Herrero L. Protocolo de investigación terapéutica con implantes osteo-integrados. Avances en Periodoncia 1992;4(3):193-195.

Schärer P, Rinn LA, Kopp FR. Principios Estéticos en la Odontología Restaurativa. Barcelona: Doyma, 1991.

Sellers GC. Direct assembly framework for osseointegrated implant prostheses. J Prosthet Dent 1989;62:662-668.

Siirila HS, Nordeberg L, Oikarinen VJ. Technique for converting an existing complete denture to a tissue-integrated prosthesis. J Prosthet Dent 1988;59:463-467.

Spector MR, Donovan TE, Nicholls JI. An evaluation of impression techniques for osseointegrated implants. J Prosthet Dent 1990;63:444-447.

Stewart RB, Desjardins R, Laney WR, Chao EYS. Fatigue strength of cantilevered metal frameworks for tissue-integrated prostheses. J Prosthet Dent 1992;68:83-92.

Thompson WP, Grohman KM, Liao R. Bonding of adhesive resins to nonprecious alloys [abstract 1258]. J Dent Res 1985;64:314.

van Steenberghe D. A retrospective multicenter evaluation of the survival rate of osseointegrated fixtures supporting fixed bridges in the treatment of partial edentulism. J Prosthet Dent 1989;61:217-223.

Wada T. Development of a new adhesive material and its properties. Proceedings of the International Symposium on Adhesive Prosthodontics. Academy of Dental Materials 1986:9-19.

Worthington P, Bolender CL, Taylor TD. The Swedish system of osseointegrated implants: Problems and complications encountered during a 4-year trial period. Int J Oral Maxillofac Implants 1987;2:277-284.

LABORATORY

Auguste P. Soldadura. Madrid: Paraninfo, 1984.

García Poggio JA. Aleaciones ligeras. Ingeniería Aeronáutica y Astronáutica 1989 (Dec, no. 320).

Gonzáles Vázquez J. Manual de Soldadura con Llama, ed 3. Barcelona: Ceac, 1983.

Jiménez V, Torroba P. Diseño de prótesis sobre implantes para conseguir ajuste pasivo. Actualidad Implantológica 1992;1(3):27-32.

López Alvarez JL. Técnicas de Laboratorio en Prótesis Fija. Madrid: Goya, 1987.

Nobelpharma Product Catalogue. Göteborg, Sweden: Nobelpharma AB, 1992.

Rangert B, Jemt T, Jörnéus L. Fuerza y momentos de los implantes. Avances en Odontoestomatología 1990;6(7):397-403.

Surgery   110, 200
Surgical stent   110
Syndrome
    Urban   21

T

Teeth
    Acrylic resin   17
Telescopic   94
Tomography   13
Temporal   34
Temporaries   51, 59, 92, 193
Tightener   21
Tin plating   141, 143
TMJ   22, 32
Torque control   46
Traction   155
Tray   153
Treatment   15

Trigger point   34
Tripadism   27
Try-in (mouth)   215, 220

V

Vaseline   145, 154
Vertical dimension   20, 107, 117, 121, 214, 218
    Compromised   117
    Noncompromised   107
Visco-gel   107
Visor   121

W

Wax box   118
Wax wafer   164
Working
    Condyle   24
    Single   24

CONTRIBUTORS:

Dr. Javier Alvarez Carlón
Orthodontist. Madrid, Spain

Dr. Pedro Badanelli Marcano
Endodontist. Madrid, Spain

Dr. Carlos Benito Cristóbal
Head of Dept. Neuroradiology
Hospital Gregorio Marañón. Madrid, Spain

Dr. Jose María Botella Pérez
Restorative and Esthetic Dentistry. Madrid, Spain

Dr. Juan Canut Brusola
Orthodontist. Madrid, Spain

Dr. Jaime Gil Lozano
Professor
Dept. Of Stomatology
University of the Basque Country. Bilbao, Spain

Dr. Thomas P. Keogh
Professor Dental Laboratory
T.P. Sanitary School, Pamplona, Spain

Dr. Ramón Martínez Corriá
Implant Surgeon. Madrid, Spain

Dr. Jose Manuel Navarro Alonso
Implant Surgery and Prosthodontics,
Las Palmas de Gran Canaria, Spain